Richard M. Satava · Achille Gaspari · Nicola Di Lorenzo (Eds.)

Emerging Technologies in Surgery

Richard M. Satava · Achille Gaspari
Nicola Di Lorenzo

Emerging Technologies in Surgery

With 90 Figures and 2 Tables

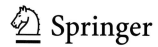 Springer

Richard M. Satava, MD
Professor of Surgery
Department of Surgery
University of Washington Medical Center
1959 NE Pacific St Rm BB487
Seattle, WA 98195
USA

Achille Gaspari, MD
Tor Vergata University of Rome
Department of General Surgery
Viale Oxford, 81
00133 Rome, Italy

Nicola Di Lorenzo, MD
Tor Vergata University of Rome
Department of General Surgery
Viale Oxford, 81
00133 Rome, Italy

Supported by: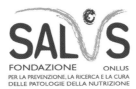

Library of Congress Control Number: 2006934463

ISBN   978-3-540-39599-7 Springer Berlin Heidelberg New York

Springer is a part of Springer Science+Business Media
springer.com

© Springer-Verlag Berlin Heidelberg 2007

Editor: Gabriele Schröder, Heidelberg, Germany
Desk Editor: Stephanie Benko, Heidelberg, Germany
Reproduction, typesetting and production: LE-TEX Jelonek, Schmidt & Vöckler GbR, Leipzig, Germany
Cover design: Frido Steinen-Broo, EStudio, Calamar, Spain

Printed on acid-free paper 24/3180/YL 5 4 3 2 1 0

Dedication

To our devoted wives,
Judith Satava, Franca Gaspari, and Fabiola di Lorenzo,
without whose encouragement and patience this would not have been possible.

During times of worry and frustration, you were there to console,
advise, and help us.

But most of all, you were our Muses, and gave us that unique inspiration
that lifts the mundane to the sublime.

For us, it was having you there to add that special sense of the aesthetic
that has made this monograph a true labor of love.

Foreword

We live in a technological age, and the practice of surgery is not exempt from this. Furthermore, predictions are that the inevitable trend in surgical practice is toward increasing dependence on high-technology equipment. Thus, *Emerging Technologies in Surgery* edited by Richard Satava, Achille Gaspari, and Nicola Di Lorenzo, is timely and appropriate. My experience with use of medical technologies together with my involvement in related research and development work over many years has led me to classify these technologies in four categories all expertly covered in this book: (1) *facilitative*—improve the efficiency of performance and reduce the degree of difficulty of execution of specific tasks; (2) *additive*—bring technical sophistication and accuracy to surgical manipulations/interventions that are not considered essential to existing practice; (3) *enabling*—make possible certain surgical interventions or open new therapeutic approaches; and (4) *disruptive*—technologies that, by breaking new ground, underpin real progress. The term "disruptive technologies" was first coined by Clayton M. Christensen in 1997 in his book *The Innovator's Dilemma* (Harvard Business School Press), to refer to technologies that, as they mature, alter the way humans live and work.

Wisely, the three editors of this book, rather than pigeonholing the technologies covered in this excellent monograph, have adopted a different layout more suited—from a practical and educational standpoint—to the current and future practice of surgery; however, examples of all these categories are included in the various sections. The contributions to all these sections are by leading-edge experts in the respective fields, and after reading all the chapters, I have no doubts that the editors chose their contributors wisely. *Emerging Technologies in Surgery* should be of interest to both the surgical trainees and their trainers, because it contains a wealth of useful and practical information on the subject. It is appropriate in my view that emphasis has been made on education and training, as they are axiomatic to quality care in surgical practice. The advances in virtual surgical simulation that, after

a shaky start, have in the last few years progressed to a stage where no surgical training program can afford to overlook their importance; the apprenticeship system of training is no longer sufficient, especially with the curtailment of the training period. The World Wide Web and progress in medical informatics in general (disruptive technologies in the extreme) have removed all possible excuses for all healthcare providers—let alone surgeons—to be misinformed or be lacking in medical up-to-date information, because the technology brings accurate information to the shop floor of medical practice. There is, however, one issue directly related to the increasing dependence of surgical care on high technology that I feel has been overlooked in all training programs and which needs emphasis: Surgeons and other interventionalists increasingly use sophisticated energized equipment often and regrettably, without an adequate understanding of the physical and engineering principles involved. This cognitive deficit of current training program needs correction.

It seems to me that the approaches covered in the various sections of *Emerging Technologies in Surgery* are breaking down turf barriers between disciplines, such that patient management is slowly changing from isolated, single-discipline treatment to multidisciplinary treatment by disease-related treatment groups, which surgeons must buy into. The spate of integrations, witnessed on both sides of the Atlantic between vascular surgeons and interventional vascular radiologists over the past 5 years, is a pertinent example.

The editors are to be congratulated for an immensely readable and informative monograph. It deserves to be read and will, I am sure, be well received. I suspect, however, that we shall witness several future editions since one thing is sure: Medical technology does not stand still ... for long.

Sir Alfred Cuschieri, FRS
Professor of Surgery
Pisa

Preface

Tremendous acceleration and changes in our daily medical practice are occurring. Both as doctors and ordinary citizens, we are aware of living in a world more and more influenced by information technology. In surgery, this revolution has brought about a dramatic acceleration of the introduction of new devices, techniques, and procedures that are changing patients' treatment and destiny. In the last 30 years, innovation has developed exponentially, forcing both current and future generations to deal with new technologies such as microsurgery or laparoscopy, and informatics. Meanwhile, the old surgical approach still needs to be learned and mastered for patients' safety.

Therefore, we decided to offer this book to illustrate to the practicing surgeon, who has precious little time to keep up with these rapid changes, what the important emerging technologies are that could affect his or her practice in the next 10–20 years. We approached this effort with the expectation that this book will serve as a useful reference to introduce surgeons of every generation to the principles of new technologies, and to familiarize them with those new procedures and de-vices that seem to belong to the future but in reality are being implemented now. Because time and resources are not infinite for the surgeon, both in everyday life and in their busy practice, we hope this monograph will contribute to their ability to select those innovations that will positively impact on his or her practice.

To that end, we have invited eminent surgeons who are experts on emerging procedures and significant advances in their respective fields to participate. We have been fortunate to assemble authors who are acknowledged authorities in these areas, both in clinical practice as well as in surgical education. We are grateful to them for their essential contributions, to bring together, outline, and illustrate the future trends. We are especially indebted to Dr. Manzelli for his invaluable support during the preparation of this work. We are proud to have the privilege to stand on the shoulders of these giants.

Richard M. Satava, Seattle
Achille L. Gaspari, Roma
Nicola Di Lorenzo, Roma

Contents

List of Contributors

Enrico Benedetti
University of Illinois at Chicago
College of Medicine
840 S. Wood Street
Suite 402, CSB (M/C 958)
Chicago, IL 60612
USA

Mark W. Bowyer MD, FACS
Uniformed Services University
of the Health Sciences
4301 Jones Bridge Road
Bethesda, MD 20814-4799
USA

Gerhard F. Bueß, MD
Section for Minimally Invasive Surgery
University of Tübingen
72072 Tübingen
Germany

Adriano De Majo
Division of General Surgery
Department of Surgery
Tor Vergata University of Rome
Viale Oxford, 81
00133 Rome
Italy

Nicola Di Lorenzo, MD
Division of General Surgery
Department of Surgery
Tor Vergata University of Rome
Viale Oxford, 81
00133 Rome
Italy

Anthony G. Gallagher, PhD
Department of Surgery
Emory University Hospital
Room B206
1364 Clifton Road, NE
Atlanta, GA 30322
USA

Timothy Ganous, MPA
University of Maryland School of Medicine
351 West Camden, CY-211
Baltimore, MD 21201
USA

Achille Lucio Gaspari, MD
Division of General Surgery
Department of Surgery
Tor Vergata University of Rome
Viale Oxford, 81
00133 Rome
Italy

Santiago Horgan, MD
Minimally Invasive Surgery
University of Illinois
840 South Wood Street
Room 435 E
Chicago, Il 60612
USA

Eiji Kanehira
Endosurgery Laboratory Kanehira (ELK)
Kanazawa
Japan

Michael S. Kavic, MD
Director of Education, General Surgery
St. Elizabeth Health Center
Professor of Clinical Surgery and Vice Chair,
Department of Surgery
Northeastern Ohio Universities College of Medicine
1044 Belmont Avenue, P.O. Box 1790
Youngstown, OH 44501-1790
USA

Antonio Manzelli, MD
Division of General Surgery
Department of Surgery
Tor Vergata University of Rome
Viale Oxford, 81
00133 Rome
Italy

Jacques Marescaux, MD, FRCS, FACS
IRCAD-EITS
1 Place de l'Hôpital
67091 Strasbourg Cedex
France

Federico Moser, MD
Minimally Invasive Surgery Center
University of Illinois
840 South Wood Street, Room 435 E
Chicago, IL 60612
USA

Didier Mutter, MD, PhD
IRCAD-EITS
1 Place de l'Hôpital
67091 Strasbourg Cedex
France

Toru Nagase
Therapeutic Products Development Department
Research & Development Division
Olympus Medical Systems Corporation
Tokyo, Japan

Jeffrey L. Ponsky, MD
Department of Surgery
Mount Sinai Medical Center
One Mount Sinai Drive
Cleveland, OH 44106
USA

Piero Rossi
Division of General Surgery
Department of Surgery
Tor Vergata University of Rome
Viale Oxford, 81
00133 Rome
Italy

Richard M. Satava, MD FACS
Professor of Surgery
Department of Surgery
University of Washington Medical Center
1959 NE Pacific St Rm BB487
Seattle, WA   98195
USA

and

Advanced Biomedical Technologies Program
Defense Advanced Research Projects Agency
Arlington, Virginia
USA

and

Telemedicine and Advanced Technology
Research Center (TATRC)
US Army Military Research and Materiel
Command (USAMRMC)*
Ft. Detrick, Maryland
USA

Michael Shin, PhD
Department of Surgery
Massachusetts General Hospital
and Harvard Medical School
55 Fruit Street
Boston, MA 02114-2696
USA

Marc O. Schurr, MD
IHCI Institute
Steinbeis University Berlin
Gürtelstraße 29A/30
10247 Berlin
Germany

J. Sutherland, MD
University of Maryland
School of Medicine
351 West Camden, CY-211
Baltimore, MD 21201, USA

Joseph P. Vacanti, MD
Department of Surgery
Massachusetts General Hospital
and Harvard Medical School
55 Fruit Street
Boston, MA 02114-2696, USA

Amy E. Waitman, MD
St. Elizabeth Health Center
Department of Surgery
1044 Belmont Avenue
Youngstown, OH 44505, USA

Masahiro Waseda, MD
Section for Minimally Invasive Surgery
University of Tübingen
72072 Tübingen, Germany

Part I
Introduction

Overview of Emerging Technologies

1

Achille Lucio Gaspari and Antonio Manzelli

Around 20 years ago, few had been able to imagine the future of surgery. Scientific progress and potentiality are amazing, and the next century will proceed in a radical new approach towards the practice of medicine. It will be based on information technology, defined as the devices that acquire information; those that process, transmit, and distribute information, and those that use information to provide therapy. Although conventional surgery will continue to have a presence, there will be radically different surgical approaches and technologies that may become the predominant form of surgery [1]. The field of surgery is entering a time of great change, spurred on by remarkable recent advances in surgical and computer technology. Surgical robotics is on the cusp of revolutionizing evolution of the new technologies. The last decades have seen robots appearing in the operative room worldwide. Thanks to its advancement, robot technology is now regularly used in endoscopic surgery and, in general terms, in minimally invasive surgery. It is still hard to believe that the future of robotics surgery is now. The use of robots has assumed a principle role in main surgical procedures in chief medical referral centers in Western countries. It is used widely for many minimally invasive procedures including Nissen fundoplication for treatment of gastroesophageal reflux disease, radical prostatectomy, hysterectomy, donor nephrectomy for kidney transplant, and reconstruction of the kidney and ureter, producing safe and notable results with benefit for patients: smaller incisions, less injury to surrounding tissues, lower risk for wound infection, shorter hospitalizations, and quicker recoveries [2–4].

One reason surgical applications are progressing quickly is the large technology base that has been developed in robotics research in the past three decades [5]. Results in mechanical design, kinematics, control algorithms, and programming that were developed for industrial robots are directly applicable to many surgical applications. Robotics researchers have also worked to enhance robotic capabilities through adaptability (the use of sensory information to respond to changing conditions) and autonomy (the ability to carry out tasks without human supervision). The resulting sensing and interpretation techniques that are proving useful in surgery include methods for image processing, spatial reasoning and planning, and real-time sensing and control [6]. In surgery, the robotics system enhances the surgeon's precision and capabilities in laparoscopic procedures, which are performed through tiny incisions with pencil-thin instruments and cameras. The robot moves high-speed cutting tools to perform precise incisions and safe dissection, and the system provides the surgeon a three-dimensional imaging of the operating field, giving intuitive hand movement, resulting in significant improvements over standard laparoscopic surgery. We must not forget that traditional laparoscopic surgery has two-dimensional imaging, and the movement of instruments is "counterintuitive", i.e., similar to doing surgery while looking into a mirror [7].

Robotic surgical systems provide the surgeon with nearly all of the natural movements of the human wrist. They also eliminate natural hand tremors and improve dexterity to enable surgeons to do ever-finer surgery in a more controlled manner [8].

However, humans still are superior at integrating diverse sources of information, using qualitative information and exercising judgment. Humans have unexcelled dexterity and hand–eye coordination, as well as a finely developed sense of touch. Unlike interaction with robots, interaction with human members of a surgical team for instruction and explanation is straightforward. These differences in capabilities mean that current robots are restricted to simple procedures, and humans must provide detailed commands, using preoperative planning systems or by providing explicit move-by-move instructions. Even in the most sophisticated systems, robots are specialized to specific tasks within procedures; humans must prepare the patient, make many of the incisions and sutures, and perform many other functions. Robotic systems are best described as "extending human capabilities" rather than "replacing human surgeons".

In fact, what we today call robot is in reality an effector, a material performer, a transducer of a commands that are directly imparted by the human being that checks and directs closely the sensibility, the movement, and in practice therefore the action. Nevertheless, in the common imaginary the robot replaces the human being in the working assignments not as ungrateful persons, perfectly adherent to the etymology of the Czech term *robota*, or "servitude" or "forced labor". Therefore, the trick to imagining the future of surgery is really to think of robots as animated, i.e., an operator and worker endowed with artificial intelligence and founded on the development of complex neural networks to the service of human beings through a truth and height remote control.

Medicine of the future and progresses in new technologies applied to surgery is not only concept of robotics systems and their application in operating room of the future, but also diffusion of knowledge, sharing of ideas, standardization of the procedures, scientific competences of sectors, standardization of the therapies, professional and formative education that, translated in different terms, produce qualitative improvement of healthcare systems worldwide. The scenario of the world of surgery is already changing, passing from the structural organizations to reach the arena of the teaching and the future of new generations of the surgeons.

The introduction on minimally invasive surgery has demonstrated the need for training surgical skills outside the operating room, using animal model or simulators. As laparoscopic surgery involves displaying images on a screen, virtual reality simulation of surgical task is feasible. Different types of simulators have become available. All simulators aim at training psychomotor skills, and some simulators also allow training in decision making and anatomical orientation. In the near future virtual reality simulators may become a tool for training and validation of surgical skills and monitoring the training progress [9].

Another field of application of the complex world of advancement in scientific technical progress is the access and the fruition of communication. Widely present in the normal daily life of everyone—especially in Western countries—the new means and modalities of communication and information technologies have significantly revolutionized access to surgical education. The introduction of the Internet information highway into mainstream clinical practice as an information-sharing medium offers a wide range of opportunities to healthcare professional. An amazing example of a world virtual university is WebSurg.com, dedicated to minimally invasive surgery laparoscopic surgery updating and professional education, assuring contributions to the worldwide diffusion of scientific information in an easy and user-friendly way. [10].

The exponential growth in information technology is resulting in a rapid increase in the ability to develop useful applications on the Internet. It is becoming difficult for surgeons to reach their full potential unless they exploit Internet-based activities. This is because the ability to rapidly capture information of quality is an essential ingredient in a reflective approach to surgical problems. More futuristic is the prospect of using computer-based technology to operate on patients from a distance, as proposed by telesurgery. With the advent of laparoscopic surgery, a method characterized by a surgeon's lack of direct contact with the patient's organs and tissue and the availability of magnified video images, it has become possible to incorporate computer and robotic technologies into surgical procedures. Computer technology has the ability to enhance, compress, and transmit video signals and other information over long distances. These technical advances have had a profound effect on surgical procedures and on the surgeons themselves because they are changing the way surgery is taught [11].

Finally, a mention of telementoring. It is used when an experienced surgeon assists or directs another less experienced surgeon who is operating at a distance. Two- and three-dimensional, video-based laparoscopic procedures are an ideal platform for real-time transmission and thus for applying telementoring to surgery. The images viewed by the operating surgeon can easily be transmitted to a central "telesurgical mentor" and permit intraoperative interaction. Several studies have demonstrated the practicality, effectiveness, and safety of surgical telementoring. The goal of this application of telemedicine is to improve surgical education and training, expand patient care, and improve healthcare delivery by allowing access to surgical specialists. Eventually, surgical telementoring could assist in the provision of surgical care to underserved areas, and potentially facilitate the teaching of advanced surgical skills worldwide [12].

What future awaits us? Will surgeons be able to follow the entire and complex world of scientific progresses? Are surgeon of tomorrow ready to be abreast of the increase of knowledge and request of quality of assistance? Modern surgery is relatively young, and despite this it has a history noble, and illustrious sort of audacity, rush and grandiose, and perspective vision of the future. The exponential growth of unknown affairs is still intimately tied to the nature of man and the drive to attain knowledge. The future requires preparation and attention to understanding of the knowledge necessary in the exclusive direction of the interest of humanity, improving performances, increasing quality solutions, providing availability of the scientific competences of sector, standardizing procedures, and providing worldwide formative education.

References

1. Satava RM, Jones SB (1998) Laparoscopic surgery: transition to the future. Urol Clin North Am 25:93–102

2. Horgan S, Vanuno D (2001) Robots in laparoscopic surgery. J Laparoendosc Adv Surg Tech A 11:415–419

3. Hazey JW, Melvin WS (2004) Robot-assisted general surgery. Semin Laparosc Surg 11:107–112

4. Cuschieri A, Buess G, Perissat J (1992) Operative manual of endoscopic surgery. Springer, Berlin Heidelberg New York

5. Khatib O (ed) (1992) Robotics review 2. MIT Press, Cambridge, Massachusetts

6. Craig JJ (1989) Introduction to robotics: mechanics and control, 2nd edn. Addison-Wesley, Reading, Massachusetts

7. Hubens G, Coveliers H, Balliu L, Ruppert M, Vaneerdeweg W (2003) A performance study comparing manual and robotically assisted laparoscopic surgery using the da Vinci. Surg Endosc 17:1595–1599

8. Gerhardus D (2005) Robot-assisted surgery: the future is here. J Healthc Manag 48:242–251

9. Korndorffer JR Jr, Dunne JB, Sierra R, Stefanidis D, Touchard CL, Scott DJ (2005) Simulator training for laparoscopic suturing using performance goals translates to the operating room. J Am Coll Surg 201:23–29

10. Lunca S, Maisonneuve H, Marescaux J (2004) WebSurg and the Virtual University. Rev Med Chir Soc Med Nat Iasi 108:230–233. Review

11. Marescaux J, Rubino F (2003) Telesurgery, telementoring, virtual surgery, and telerobotics. Curr Urol Rep 4:109–113. Review

12. Rosser JC Jr, Herman B, Giammaria LE (2003) Telementoring. Semin Laparosc Surg 10:209–217. Review

Economics of New Surgical Technologies

2

Michael S. Kavic and Amy E. Waitman

2.1 Technology: A Definition of Terms

Technology is that body of knowledge available to a civilization that is of use in fashioning implements, practicing manual arts and skills, and extracting or collecting materials [1]. It is the science that concerns itself with the application of knowledge to practical purposes. Others have suggested that the characterization of technology be expanded to include those technologies that *sustain* the way a thing is done or performed, and those technologies that *change* the way things are accomplished [2]. In this sense, sustaining technologies are those technologies that keep up or improve the status quo but do not disrupt or create chaos in existing situations. New growth is not fostered. On the other hand, disruptive technologies are those technologies that create major new growth in areas they penetrate and disrupt or cause to fail the entrenched technologies. New growth can occur because less skilled persons are enabled to do things previously done only by expensive specialists in centralize (typically inconvenient) locations. The consumer is offered services or products that are cheaper, better, and more convenient than previously provided.

2.2 A Brief History of Medical Technology

Surgical technology and the skills to practice operative intervention were essentially embryonic for the first several thousand years of recorded history. The overwhelming and intense pain associated with surgery limited operative procedures to only those that were simple and rapid. In addition, there was limited knowledge of the role of bacteria in the development of infection. Wound contamination was common, and sepsis frequently resulted in death of the surgical patient.

The discovery of anesthesia and the acceptance of antisepsis stimulated the development of surgical instrumentation during the late 19th century. Growth, nevertheless, was slow, and technological innovation was essentially a sustaining one as clamps, retractors, scalpels, and other devices developed before or during the 19th century were refined, but little changed. Creative surgical innovators focused on ways to extirpate or correct disease processes, and new, innovative operative procedures were developed. However, the technology utilized to perform these operations remained unchanged. And remained so for almost a century. In a similar vein, costs for surgical instruments (technology) remained stable and relatively predictable.

During the latter part of the 20th and the beginning of the 21st century, however, surgery became a technology-driven profession. There was a disruption of the status quo. The development of new technologies (energy sources, mechanical devices, imaging, etc.) ultimately led to a radical change in how surgery was practiced. Spectacular medical achievements were due to advances in technology that in many instances was disruptive of the status quo. These technological advances enabled physicians to diagnose and treat disease more accurately than before. Computerized tomography (CT), magnetic resonance imaging (MRI), and diagnostic radioisotope studies revolutionized the field of radiology. Portable, affordable ultrasound units gave the gynecologist an office-based tool to accurately and conveniently diagnose female genital tract disease. Minimally invasive surgery (a stunning example of the combination of several disruptive technologies) combined solid-state cameras, high-resolution video monitors, and laparoscopes to completely change the way physicians exposed and managed surgical disease. No longer was a large traumatic surgical incision required to visualize intracavitary organs.

Present-day technologies have allowed clinicians to gather more information and refine differential diagnosis prior to operative intervention. CT scans and diagnostic laparoscopies in many instances have replaced the need for exploratory laparotomy. The result has been a decrease in patient risk and morbidity. New technologies have not only enhanced quality of life, but also in many instances, extended it.

2.3   The Economic Burden of Health Care

Men and women throughout the world and particularly in developed Western countries have come to expect, indeed to demand, high-technology health care. The advances in technology and medical devices, however, have come at a very high price and have generated wrenching ethical and social debates. National health expenditure in the United States, for example, increased from $41.0 billion, or 5.7% of the gross domestic product (GDP) in 1965, to $1,299.5 billion in 2000, or 13.2% of the GDP. National health care expenditure on a per capita basis increased from $205 in 1965 to $4,672 in 2000 [3]. Health care spending continued to rise in the United States, reaching $1.4 trillion in 2001. This was an 8.7% increase from the year 2000. Health care spending increased three times faster than did growth of the US economy. In the year 2000, health care spending was $4,672 per person, which increased to $5,035 per person in 2001 [4].

The number of medical schools in the United States increased from 86 in 1960 to 126 in 1994, and the number of medical students increased from 30,288 in 1960 to 66,629 in 1994. There were 5,407 hospitals in the United States in 1960, with 639,000 beds, and 5,321 hospitals, with 923,000 beds in 1992. Only a modest increase of hospital beds, but on the other hand, the number of freestanding ambulatory surgical centers increased from 459 in 1985 (783,864 procedures performed) to 1,862 in 1993 (3,197,956 procedures performed) [5]. The US population in 1960 was 179,323,175 people, and by the year 2001 increased to 284,796,887. Most could afford health care. As reported by the US Census Bureau in 2001, the number of persons with health insurance was 240.9 million; the number of uninsured persons was 41.2 million [6].

The increase in health care demand and supply has not been confined to the United States. All major developed countries have experienced a similar increase. For example, health care expenditures in the United Kingdom increased as a percentage of gross domestic product from 4.5% in 1970 to 7.1% in 1992. Viewed another way, this translated to health care spending per capita increase in the United Kingdom from $146 in 1970 to $1,213 in 1993. Similarly, health care spending as a percentage of gross national product in France increased from 5.8% in 1970 to 9.4% in 1992. On a per capita basis, French health care spending increased from $192 in 1970 to $1,835 in 1993. Countries in the Far East have not been exempt from this trend and in Japan, the percentage of expenditures on health care as related to gross domestic product increased from 4.4% in 1970 to 6.9% in 1992. Put another way, health care spending per capita in Japan increased from $126 in 1970 to $1,495 in 1993 [5].

The demand for health care has been fueled in part by readily available worldwide communication. Nearly universal access to mass communication, radio, television, and the Internet has educated consumers and has helped create a demand for cutting-edge care. A consensus appears to be developing that people of the world are beginning to expect certain rights of their governments including respect of person, dignity, and access to health care. Because of this public demand for health care, a major issue undergoing debate in various countries has been whether a society or a nation should restrain advances in expensive health care technology or attempt to fulfill the universal human desire for good health regardless of cost. Many believe that no one should be denied access to health care because of cost, but few deny the overwhelming importance of prudent economic management in the delivery of health care.

Costs for health care have unrelentingly spiraled upward, and there appears to be no end to the increasing financial burden on individuals, societies, and states. Demand has outstripped supply. As a benchmark, it is worth noting that the average US general surgeon performed 398 procedures per year from 1995 to 1997. Of these cases, 102 (26%) were abdominal procedures, 63 (16%) were for alimentary tract procedures, 55 (14%) were for breast operations, 51 (13%) were for endoscopic procedures, 48 (12%) cases involved soft-tissue operations, 39 (12%) cases were vascular procedures, trauma accounted for 6 (2%) cases, 4 (1%) cases were for endocrine disease, and 3 (1%) were for head and neck. Of the 398 procedures, 44 (11%) cases were for minimally invasive laparoscopic operations [7]. This is an average yearly workload for a general surgeon in the United States, and may be taken as a baseline for what a general surgeon can accomplish in a developed Western country that has a high demand for health care.

2.4   A Technological Solution to Health Care Cost

In many poorer countries, the ability (financial remuneration, personal growth, safety, quality of life issues, academic satisfaction, etc.) to supply and deliver health care is very limited or nonexistent. The solution to the dilemma of providing health care in an environment of limited resources has been obscure, but with the use of disruptive technologies, the solution may be obtainable.

Over the last 50 years, technology has revolutionized health care, and it will likely continue to do so in the future. Technology, however, comes in many guises. It is in the application of technology and, in particular, those technologies of a more simple, convenient form, that may hold the key to reducing costs and allow medical care to be more widely available.

The experience of industry with sustaining and disruptive technologies provide clues and perhaps suggest an answer to the dilemma of providing health care in this technologically driven age. Christensen et al. have suggested that sustaining innovation (technology) is the improvement an industry creates as it introduces new and more advanced products to serve the more sophisticated customers at the high end of a market [2]. Disruptive innovations (technology) are cheaper, simpler, more convenient products or services that start by meeting the needs of less demanding customers. For example, the invention of the printing press (disruptive technology) put a large number of human copiers of books out of business. The lay public was less demanding of book producers than were the clerics and academics of the day. Texts did not need to be hand printed or illuminated in gold to provide their message. The inexpensive, portable camera developed by George Eastman a century ago disrupted the art world by virtually eliminating the need for expensive portrait artists. The invention of electrophotography by Chester Carlson in 1938 (later called xerography) revolutionized the world of printing and decreased reliance on printing professionals.

In each instance, technology, particularly cheaper, simpler, and more convenient technology, disrupted the status quo, diffused throughout society, and brought great benefit to that society. Each particular technology enabled a larger population of less skilled persons to do more of a task, in a more convenient setting, and in a less expensive manner, which previously had required more highly skilled specialists. This caused an upmarket migration of service that has proven to be an essential driver of economic progress in the industrial world [2].

Health care can be transformed in a similar manner. In fact, some parts of the health care system have already been disrupted, and a transformation of sorts is underway. Outpatient surgical centers have been established that can safely and efficiently offer operative procedures that heretofore have only been performed in high-cost hospitals. Nurse practitioners and other nonphysician clinicians can function as autonomous providers of patient care and perform many of the basic tasks of a primary care physician [8]. Specialists and specialized centers (hospitals) should not be asked, or rewarded, to carry out more simple tasks that can be performed elsewhere. Yet, perversely in the real world, many health care plans have done just that.

Several US states and some insurance plans have regulations that preclude nurse practitioners from performing simple diagnostic tests and therapeutic interventions. More highly trained physicians, in order to maintain their income stream, are forced to see patients with common, simple problems. A production line is instituted in the physician's office and office visits must, by necessity, be brief and perfunctory. Instead of an upmarket migration of services where nurse practitioners or physician assistants (with appropriate enabling technology) are permitted to manage simple problems, there is a downmarket migration of services by the physician. It is no wonder that less actual care is given, and patient dissatisfaction is increased. Less expensive personnel are not utilized to perform tasks that are within their realm to accomplish when armed with appropriate (disruptive) technology. The lessons from industry have been neglected and a fundamental engine of potential medical progress has been stifled.

To frame the health care problem more clearly, it is necessary to look at the delivery of health care in terms of systems. Human disease and its management can be categorized into several tiers of complexity, ranging from the most simple to the very intricate. In the simplest tier of disease, accurate data collection reveals an unambiguous diagnosis that can be managed with a straightforward treatment protocol of medical therapy. This disease recognition and treatment process can be described as a *rule-based* process. In the middle levels of disease complexity, no single piece of information yields a diagnosis. Rather, multiple data points suggest a diagnosis and treatment program through a process of discernment by the physician called *pattern recognition*. In the most complex disease states, the diagnosis is obscure and requires the collective experience and judgment of a team of clinicians. Multiple tests are required and the diagnosis and treatment is arrived at in a *problem-solving mode* [2].

Considering the above, it is clear that at the most simple levels of disease, a rule-based process would establish the diagnosis and dictate therapy. Medical treatment could then be initiated by well-trained nonphysician clinicians and less highly skilled physicians. Application of the rule-based process would specify a proven therapeutic strategy. Technologies are available to facilitate this process. For example, a sore throat can be evaluated by a trained nonphysician clinician; appropriate, convenient, outpatient cultures (technology) obtained; and antibiotic therapy initiated on receipt of a streptococcal infection report.

Similarly, enabling technologies such as unsophisticated, inexpensive, office-based ultrasound would allow primary care physicians to evaluate breast lumps and, if cystic, manage them conservatively. Appropriate management would be initiated without referral for costly hospital or specialist evaluation. An upward migration of service will have occurred. In a similar way, endovascular stenting in an outpatient setting has the potential to cause an upward migration of service and reduce the need for a more costly surgical team, operating rooms, and hospital stay. In all of these situations, technology can be disruptive of the status quo and result in an upmarket migration of services where less skilled persons perform procedures that are more sophisticated in a less expensive way.

The introduction of new technology is as critical in the field of medicine as it has been in industry. A good guide to the introduction of technology is found in the "Statement on Emerging Surgical Technologies and the Evaluation of Credentials" promulgated by the American College of Surgeons [9]. The position taken by the American College of Surgeons recognizes that the introduction and application of any new technology should proceed through a series of steps intended to ensure its safety, appropriateness, and cost-effectiveness. These steps or recommendations suggest that the development of new technology must be accompanied by a scientific assessment of safety, efficacy, and need. Diffusion into clinical practice requires appropriate education of surgeons and evaluation of their use of the new technology. Finally, widespread application of new technologies must be continuously assessed and compared with alternative therapies to ensure appropriateness and cost-effectiveness through outcome studies.

The guidelines of the American College of Surgeons regarding technology are reasonable and patient centered. Disruptive medical technologies exist that enable persons who are less skilled to perform tasks traditionally completed by more highly trained specialists. By allowing less highly trained and less expensive practitioners to perform more highly skilled tasks with dis-

ruptive technologic innovations, more patients can be served with safety, efficiency, and cost-effectiveness.

References

1. Berube MS (1999) Webster's II new college dictionary. Houghton Mifflin, Boston
2. Christensen C, Thomas C, Hart S (2001) The great disruption. Foreign Aff 80:2
3. US Department of Health and Human Services, Centers for Medicare & Medicaid Services (2002) National health care trends in public versus private funding, selected calendar years 1965–2000. http://www.cms.hhs.gov/researchers/pubs/datacompendium/2002/02pg14.pdf. Accessed 10 March 2003
4. US Department of Health and Human Services, Centers for Medicare & Medicaid Services (2003) Report details national health care spending increases in 2001. http://cms.hhs.gov/media/press/release.asp?Counter=693
5. Roger CM, Seward WF (1996) Socio-economic factbook for surgery, 1996–1997. American College of Surgeons, Chicago
6. US Census Bureau. Health insurance coverage: 2001. http://www.census.gov/hhes/www/hlthin01.html. Accessed 10 March 2003
7. Ritchie WP, Rhodes RS, Biester TW (1999) Work loads and practice patterns of general surgeons in the United States, 1995–1997. Ann Surg 230:533–543
8. Cooper RA, Henderson T, Dietrich CL (1998) Roles of nonphysician clinicians as autonomous providers of patient care. JAMA 280:795–802
9. American College of Surgeons (2000) Statement on emerging surgical technologies and the evaluation of credentials. http://www.facs.org/fellows_info/statements/st-18.html

The Scientific, Social, and Ethical Implications of Disruptive Technologies

3

Richard M. Satava*

Technology has been a major driver of all revolutionary change that occurs on a large scale. As we leave the Information Age and head into the next era, it is prudent to examine the extraordinary technologies that are emerging from the scientific laboratory, and to attempt to understand the social and ethical impact that these technologies would have on healthcare, society, and our species.

3.1   Introduction

In 1980, Alvin Toffler [1] described the three ages of man: the Agriculture Age, the Industrial Age, and the "new" Information Age. The purpose was to call to public attention and scrutiny what was perceived to be a new, major change in our society as a whole. This change, the Information Age, was described as a new revolution that was predicated upon a new technology that would totally change the entire fabric of daily living. The premise was that entire societies of the previous ages, the Agriculture Age and the Industrial Age, were based on a specific technology—farming, and then machines. The Information Age is based on telecommunications and computers—the dispersal of information. Agriculture societies were intent on providing survival for themselves, their families, or immediate community. With the Industrial Age, a few people were able to provide the food and material needs of thousands or millions of people by way of efficient machine technology, be it tractors and harvesters for food or mass production of clothing, transportation, and other devices. In the Information Age, rather than working directly in various goods, there was a major switch to a service industry in which people did not grow, build, or make something, but rather were intermediaries that provided other peoples' (or manufactured) products or performed service for them.

The Information Age is actually over 100 years old, including technologies such as the radio, television,

telephones, computers, and the Internet, although Toffler chooses to date it as beginning after World War II. During this Information Age, the majority of people did not farm their own food nor make any products nor even perform manual labor for someone else, but rather dealt in the intangible information. The focus is on making information available in a timely (usually rapid) manner in order to make better decisions, to acquire a market position, archive massive amounts of information for reference, to connect people with other people or information in a ubiquitous manner, etc. There is nothing substantive, no ear of corn, new clay pot, or even a hole in the ground. Instead, there are ideas, datasets, and networks. Moreover, a *chat room* is not a room but a computer program to share messages and conversation—in essence, a virtual room. The results have been to make a larger amount of information available distributed throughout the world, so fewer people could make even vaster amounts of food and products available, freeing the majority of the population to either concentrate on producing more information (away from manual labor) or more leisure time. In addition, many inanimate objects, such as telephones, automobiles, computers, and even robots started the earliest, primitive level of "intelligence". These machines and devices could do very simple tasks that people used to do. Cell phones store phone numbers, automobiles have automatic adjusting breaks, and televisions and videocassette recorders are programmable and have remote controls. Throughout these three ages or revolutions, humans have remained unchanged: What humans *do* is changed but, with the exception of a significant reduction in disease (and a resultant slight increase in living longer lives), humans are exactly physically the same as we have been in the past hundreds of thousands of years.

More important for understanding the various ages and the transitions, there comes a time when a revolution (such as the Industrial Age) goes from revolution to evolution. Figure 3.1 is a conceptual graphic of the ages. What is noticed is that there is a "tail" at

---

* The opinions or assertions contained herein are the private views of the authors and are not to be construed as official, or as reflecting the views of the Department of the Army, Department of the Navy, the Advanced Research Projects Agency, or the Department of Defense.

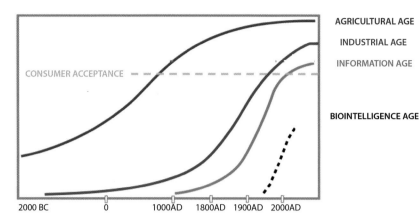

AGRICULTURAL AGE

INDUSTRIAL AGE

INFORMATION AGE

BIOINTELLIGENCE AGE

Fig. 3.1 The ages of the development of technology

the beginning of the revolution, which shows a small amount of change in the new technology: discovery. A point is reached when there is a very rapid growth of the new technology: commercialization. The "revolution" is now taken by society as a whole, for example Henry Ford making the automobile available to everyone: consumer acceptance. Any subsequent changes in the technology are evolutionary rather than revolutionary. Once a revolution has achieved consumer acceptance, any subsequent changes that are made are iterative, making the product better but not inventing a new product. The rapid growth in technology flattens out and no significant new technology is invented. It appears that this plateau effect has been achieved with Information Age technologies, as manifest by the ubiquitous use of cell phones, computers, the Internet, etc. There has not been a new invention in information technology in over a decade; the researchers are simply making the things we have better or cleverer. If there are no "new and revolutionary technologies" being created by Information Age technologies, then in what direction and with what technology will the next revolution occur?

There appears to be another new age occurring. Because this is the very middle of change, it is hard to perceive the trends and interpret the essence of the change around us, and it is not possible to prove that a change is occurring, so the following speculation is offered. In looking at Fig. 3.1, there is a new tail represented that has not reached the "Consumer Acceptance Line". This trend is rooted in the discoveries in biology over the past 30 to 50 years, and not only in the discovery of DNA and the Human Genome, but also in the many pharmaceuticals and consumer products based on biological principles. In addition, the primordial efforts during the Information Age at making devices intelligent are now expanding exponentially. The Information Age bar codes have made all products identifiable all the time, linked to many important functions

for stores, and so on. Credit cards provide access at all times to all things that can be purchased, either directly or via the Internet. But new microtechnologies such as the radio frequency identification (RFID) tags are complete computers that are so tiny (smaller than the head of a pin) that virtually everything from food to clothes to appliances will have a tiny bit of intelligence embedded inside and will be able to communicate with one another. The result is a world in which even inanimate objects are "smarter", and they "talk" with one another. Perhaps this could be considered the first step toward a new life form, one capable of communicating by itself but not "living" in the same sense as do people. But most importantly, this revolution is being led not by individual brilliant researchers discovering something in their tiny niche, but rather by large, interdisciplinary teams that have expertise in many areas, with a heavy emphasis on biologic sciences. The discovery and understanding of the complexity of the world has progressed to the point where no single person can understand the truly large issues, and any fundamentally revolutionary change can only be achieved by interdisciplinary teams. The term "BioIntelligence Age" [2] has been proposed as a placeholder name for this new direction, because it illustrates the combination of the importance of the discoveries in biology, physical sciences, and information sciences (Fig. 3.2). Discoveries are occurring at the interface of two or more of the technologies, creating something that a single discipline could not develop alone.

On this broad background, it is appropriate to investigate how one portion of this change in science and technology—healthcare—is accommodating to the future. Although many of the technologies that will affect the future are being discovered in the basic sciences, their ultimate use will be for health care purposes, or require implementation by a health care provider. The technologies to be addressed have been chosen because of the profound questions they raise for individ-

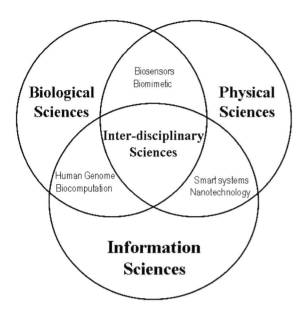

Fig. 3.2 The BioIntelligence Age, and ages of interdisciplinary research

uals, society, and the species as a whole. While many have been considered as being in the realm of science fiction, recent discoveries have been subjected to the rapid acceleration of technology and therefore will appear much earlier than anticipated: Science fiction will soon become scientific fact! These new discoveries will launch the moral and ethical challenges that today's students and residents must solve during their careers.

3.2 Intelligent Computers and Robots

The human brain has been estimated to compute at the speed of 4×10^{19} computations per second (cps) [3]. The latest supercomputer, Red Storm at Los Alamos National Laboratories (Los Alamos, N.M), computes at 4×10^{15} cps, still about 1,000 times slower than the human brain computes. However, Moore's Law (roughly interpreted as "computer power doubles every 18 months") would indicate that computers will be as fast (or faster) than humans are in 15–20 years. New programming techniques, such as genetic algorithms, cellular automata, neural networks, etc., are designed to "learn", The result will be computers, machines, and robots with greater computing power than humans, and that will have the ability to learn from experience, to adapt to new or novel situations, and design a solution to new situations. Will they be intelligent? Will humans "communicate" with them? If they are intel-

ligent, are they "alive" and must they be given "rights?" Will they even remember that we created them, or even care?

3.3 Human Cloning

There exist numerous human clones in many different countries, with publications about them coming from China, Korea, and Italy [4]. The United States and most of the world community has banned human cloning. Was that a prudent move or just a knee-jerk reaction? With an ever-escalating world population and millions of starving people, why is it necessary to clone a human? Although there has not been a formal conclusion on how to address the issue of human cloning, it is banned in most countries. Was that a correct decision, or should a family that has tried all known forms of medical reproduction and failed be given a chance to have their own child through cloning? Is cloning one more step in the "natural" evolution of humans?

3.4 Genetic Engineering

The first genetically engineered child was born in 2003 to a family with three boys. The parents decided to "engineer" their fourth child to be a girl; this and many other examples are discussed by Gregory Stock in his book *Redesigning Humans: Our Inevitable Genetic Future* [5]. Not only is it possible to choose through engineering specific favorable human traits, but also genetic sequences for a number of diseases have been studied, and there are children who have had the disease trait engineered out in order to have a normal, happy life. Other parents have chosen to use genetic engineering for a second child (the "survivor sibling") when the firstborn child develops an incurable disease (like leukemia) [6]. The newborn child's normal hemopoetic stem cells can provide a rejection-free replenishment for the firstborn who has had total irradiation of bone marrow to cure the leukemia. Is it moral to specifically engineer and conceive one child in order to save another?

Another aspect of genetic engineering is that the genetic sequences for specific traits in one species (e.g., genes that allow reptiles and hummingbirds to see in the dark with infrared or ultraviolet vision [7, 8]) are well characterized and have been successfully transplanted across species. Should humans be engineering their children, not only with traits to make them better or stronger humans, but also with traits that go beyond known human capabilities such as the infrared vision and others, especially if the new trait provides an important new advantage? How will it be decided who can receive such genetic traits that give a person a superior advantage?

3.5   Longevity

The longest recorded human lifespan is 123 years. One of the major determinants in longevity is the telomere on a chromosome—when a cell divides, the telomere is shortened by the enzyme telomerase, eventually resulting in a telomere that is too short to sustain further division and hence, the cell dies. There are a few strains of mice (and "immortal" cell lines) that have been engineered to produce antitelomerase, which blocks the enzyme telomerase and maintains the length of the telomere; these mice are able to live two to three times a normal life span [9]. If this mechanism is also effective in humans, should we do human trials to determine if a person can live 200 years, or longer? If longevity is successful, what are the social implications of living 200 years? Does the person retire at 60 years of age, with 140 years of retirement? How would it be possible for the planet to support the massive increase in population if people could live so long?

3.6   Human–Machine Communication

A number of centers around the world now have implanted probes into monkeys' brains and read the signals when a monkey moves its arms to feed itself [10]. By training the monkey to eat, and then decoding these signals, it has been possible to send the signals for eating directly to a robotic arm. In a short time, the monkey is able to feed itself with the robotic arm simply by thinking of feeding itself. Where can this technology lead? To putting probes in the brain to directly connect to a computer or the Internet? As the control of artificial limbs and other parts of the body becomes more successful, should these limb prostheses be used to replace those of paraplegics or quadriplegics? Will such persons be true cyborgs (half human–half machine)?

3.7   Artificial Organs and Prostheses

The following example typifies the interdisciplinary approach needed to achieve success in designing and creating complex living systems, such as growing artificial organs to replace diseased organs. The following illustration approximates the system pioneered by Dr. Joseph Vacanti [11] of Massachusetts General Hospital (MGH) and Massachusetts Institute of Technology (MIT), and is described in order to understand the critical need for an interdisciplinary approach in research and healthcare. Using computational mathematics, a complete microvascular system with an artery and vein that anastomoses at a 10-μm size (red blood cells are 8 μm in size) is computer designed. This design is exported to a stereolithography machine (a 3-D printer) that "prints" this blood vessel system, using a bioresorbable polymer designed by chemists in which angiogenesis factor, platelet-derived growth factor, and other cell growth promoters from molecular biologists are embedded. This artificial scaffold is then suspended in a bioreactor (a bath with fluid that supports cell growth), to which is added vascular endothelial stem cells. The stem cells grow and absorb the scaffold, leaving a living microvascular system; this is placed into another bioreactor with hepatic stem cells, and a miniature liver is grown while the blood vessels are perfused. The result is a tiny portion of a synthetically grown liver, which is able to support growth and can produce the products (albumen, globulin, etc.) a natural liver would produce. The challenge for the future is to test if this will survive when implanted in an animal, and whether it will be able to scale up to a full human-size liver grown from a person's own stem cells. There are a number of alternate approaches as well. Using a printed matrix of substrate to attract promote natural stem cell growth; a stereolithograph printer that can print a number of different cell types simultaneously to print an entire organ; and transgenic pigs that can grow an organ that is not rejected by a human, as well as other innovations are being investigated. With such a large amount of research from many different approaches, it is highly likely that in the near future synthetically grown organs will be available on demand.

Another successful technique for designing replacement parts for humans is that of intelligent prostheses. While current orthopedic prostheses, such as hips and other joints, have been successful for decades, re-replacement is often needed because of wear from mechanical stress and strain, fracturing, etc. New research includes microsensors and actuators into prostheses, which can then respond to the stresses and adjust the prosthesis to take the strain off the bone and provide for a more stable and longer-lived prosthesis, or implantable micropumps that can sense blood sugar levels and release insulin to control diabetes [12]. As development continues in synthetic (living) or prosthetic replacement parts for humans, it may be possible to replace most of the human body with synthetics (cyborg). Will there be a threshold reached when a person is more than 90% synthetic replacements, and if so, will that person still be "human?" What exactly is it

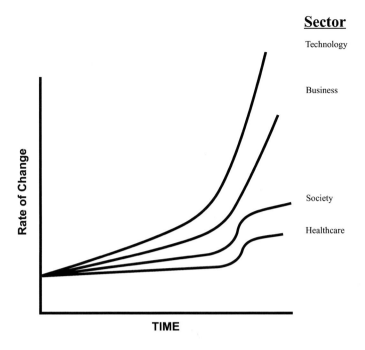

Sector

Technology

Business

Society

Healthcare

Fig. 3.3 The rate of change in different sectors in response to disruptive technology

that determines being human? Is it the flesh and blood with which a person is born?

3.8 Suspended Animation

The research at the University of Alaska, Fairbanks, of hibernation has elucidated some key knowledge: Animals do not hibernate because it is cold; they hibernate because they control their metabolism and literally "turn off" their need for oxygen [13]. The evidence for the mechanism of action is postulated to be signaling molecules that arise in the hypothalamus and attach to the mitochondrial membrane, preventing oxidative phosphorylation. In a complementary fashion, Safar et al., at the University of Pittsburg Center for Resuscitation Research [14], have a reproducible animal model in which they can exsanguinate the animal to a point where there is no blood pressure, respiration, or electroencephalographic activity (clinical death) and perfuse the animal with a hypothermic perfusate. Two hours later, the shed blood is reinfused, the animal regains consciousness, and 2 weeks later meets all criteria of normal, including cognitive function. These and similar projects provide the scientific basis for significant progress toward suspended animation. Will suspended animation replace anesthesia? If there is success in suspended animation for more than a few hours, days, years, or decades, what are the consequences for society? Should all people with terminal diseases be placed in suspended animation until a cure for their disease

is found? What happens when a person is suspended for decades and awakes in the future, e.g., financially, psychologically, etc.? Will only a few persons be able to afford this treatment?

3.9 Summary

The future is bright with disruptive technologies, and the rate at which such technology is being developed is accelerating logarithmically (Fig. 3.3). Technology development explodes with a revolutionary scientific breakthrough, and business is close behind with commercialization plans to profit from the new technology. However, society is much slower to respond, especially in addressing many of the moral and ethical issues raised above. The medical profession is even slower to respond; there needs to be stringent evaluation and validation to ensure the new discovery is safe and applicable to patients. The medical profession is caught between two conflicting priorities: not providing a new diagnostic modality or treatment quickly enough, and not jumping on every bandwagon before the science is proven safe and effective for patients (*primum non nocerum)*. The other aspect of the rapid scientific development is a society that is not prepared to deal quickly with the enormous psychological changes, at both the societal and individual person levels.

The technologies above are discussed in greater depth in many scientific discourses, as well as in the following chapters; however, there has been very little attention to the consequences of the innovation, either intended or unintended. These technologies are revolutionary and will take decades to become commonplace. Likewise, the moral and ethical issues raised by these disruptive changes will take decades to debate and resolve [15]. Now is the time to begin consideration and debate; if we wait, as in the case of human cloning, the science will overtake our ability to respond. And the issues to be addressed are so much more fundamental than they were in the past, when the focus was on an individual or society. Some of the technologies challenge our most basic tenants, such as what it means to be human, should we design our children, can machines become human and have rights, and even, what *is* evolution? With these new powers from science, the moral and ethical consequences are even more threatening. For the first time in history, there now walks upon this planet a species so powerful that it can create its own evolution to its own choosing: *Homo sapiens.* What shall humans choose to become?

References

1. Toffler A (1980) The third wave. Bantam, New York, pp 8–12

2. Satava RM (ed.) (2000) Innovative technologies: the Information Age and the BioIntelligence Age. Surg Endosc 14:417–418

3. Kurzweil R (2000) The Age of Spiritual Machines. Penguin Putnam, New York, pp 102–104

4. Hwang WS, Ryu YJ, Park JH et al (2004) Evidence of a pluripotent human embryonic stem cell line derived from a cloned blastocyst. Science doi:10.1126 /science.1094515

5. Stock G (2002) Redesigning humans: our inevitable genetic future. Houghton Mifflin, New York

6. Verlinsky Y, Rechitsky S, Sharapova T, Morris R, Taranissi M, Kuliev A (2004) Preimplantation HLA testing. JAMA 29:2079

7. Gorbunov V, Fuchigami N, Stone M, Grace M, Tsukruk VV (2002) Biological thermal detection: micromechanical and microthermal properties of biological infrared receptors. Biomacromolecules 3:106–115

8. Goldsmith TH (1980) Hummingbirds see near ultraviolet light. Science 207:786–788

9. Saito K, Yoshioka H, Cutler RG (1998) A spin trap, *N-tert-*butyl-α-phenylnitrone extends the life span of mice. Biosci Biotechnol Biochem 62:792–794

10. Serruya MD, Hatsopolous NG, Paninski L, Fellows MR, Donoghue JP (2002) Brain–machine interface: instant neural control of a movement signal. Nature 416:141

11. Lalan S, Pomerantsva I, Vacanti JP (2001) Tissue engineering and its potential impact on surgery. World J Surg 25:1458–1466

12. Selam JL (2001) External and implantable insulin pumps: current place in the treatment of diabetes. Exp Clin Endocrinol Diabetes 109(Suppl 2): S333–S340

13. Buck CL, Barnes BM (2000) Effects of ambient temperature on metabolic rate, respiratory quotient, and torpor in an arctic hibernator. Am J Physiol 279:R255–R262

14. Safar P, Ebmeyer U, Katz L, Tisherman S (eds) (1996) Future directions for resuscitation research. Crit Care Med 24(Suppl 2):S1–S99

15. Fukyama F (2002) Our post-human future: consequence of the biotechnology revolution. Farrar, Straus and Giroux, New York

Part II
Education and Training

The World Virtual University and the Internet: http://www.websurg.com

4

Jacques Marescaux and Didier Mutter

The WebSurg World Virtual University originates from the success of the Institute for Research into Cancer of the Digestive System (Institut de Recherche contre les Cancers de l'Appareil Digestif [IRCAD]) International School of Surgery. The concept of this school is to unify academic teaching and tutorials delivered by international experts able to share and confront their opinions about the most recent approaches in laparoscopic surgery. To overcome the geographical constraints of the school located in Strasbourg, France, we had to envision an original way of reproducing this concept and make it available anywhere in the world, with no time and access restrictions whatsoever: The Internet stood out as the solution.

The new means and modalities of communication and information technologies have significantly revolutionized the access to surgical education. The introduction of the Internet information highway into mainstream clinical practice as an information-sharing medium offers many opportunities to healthcare professionals. The Internet favors an easy, worldwide diffusion of scientific information. As a result, daily surgical practice shows an increase in the use of the Internet to gather, transform, and disseminate surgical data.

In earlier years, access to information was primarily done through paper (journals, books, etc.). The impact of the Internet on information diffusion is indirectly confirmed by the irritation of the traditional book publishers facing the intent of Google, one of the major Internet providers, to digitize and index the library collections of major research universities [1]. The Internet, with its capacity to federate all networks, is progressively superseding all other education media. In addition, the Internet appeals to the surgical community with its main characteristics, i.e., interactivity, multimedia user-friendliness, and quick access to and low cost of information. This cybermedicine allows sharing of data with an unlimited number of Web users including patients or industrialists. The notion of universal information exchange represents the benefit of the Internet, based on sharing of information. Each user may find his or her field of interest in the wide range of data available. Since nowadays almost every physician is connected to the Internet, and thanks to the quality of specific search engines specialized in medical publications such as PubMed or ones more generic such as Google, surgeons have the ability to use the Internet in their practices. The surgical community can easily find extensive theoretical and practical information that may be used in order to acquire, test, and validate new operative skills from any geographical location in the world. Physicians, and especially surgeons, spend a considerable amount of time in educational activities. It is confirmed by the growing number of continuing medical education (CME) credit points delivered each year through educational websites (approximately 10% of all delivered CME credit points) [2].

Both surgeons and information providers (universities as well as the industry) quickly understood the attraction of virtual learning and its convenience. The Internet allows independent work whenever and wherever possible. Online information is available everywhere, 24 hours a day, and 7 days a week, with no constraints of time or space. In this respect, surgeons may continue to provide care for patients while improving their knowledge and practice skills. Additionally, they may remain connected to their favorite website and concentrate on surgical indications, or watch videos and descriptions of conventional or new surgical procedures.

A recent search performed on Google using generic keywords like "education" and "surgery" listed more than 9,800,000 websites (Table 4.1). The extraordinary amount of websites found there represent not only reputable educational information but also millions of websites run by individuals, business, advocacy groups, and clubs, serving different intentions and audiences. Sorting out such a massive amount of material, one kernel of medical information often appears to be frustrating. The frustration raised and unreliability of certain sources of information drove some surgeons to develop high-quality, specialized, and dedicated websites. Thanks to such specialization, online educational activity is gaining more and more acceptance [3]. To support this evidence, a survey was recently administered by Gandsas et al. [3] to members of the Society of American Gastro-Intestinal Endoscopic Surgeons (SAGES). Respondents were recruited to participate through a mass e-mailing or by visiting www.laparoscopy.com. In this study, 78% of the respondents used the Internet to expand their knowledge of surgery, 74% to learn about the technologies related to the practice of surgery, and 68% to locate resources for academic purposes. The power and potency of these dedicated websites is directly correlated with their quality. We developed an original multimedia website, www.websurg.com, whose contents are written by surgeons under the control and seal of approval of national and international scientific societies (Fig. 4.1).

The prerequisites for success have been met: a technological quality with a real use of multimedia and, notably, video streaming techniques may be observed. There is also a respect for cultural diversity, and reliability. Quality is the key factor for success in the long term, even though its price may be high. Quality means having the best, most renowned authors whose content of their chapters and videos must be checked and approved of by a peer review committee. The peer review process seems to offer a guarantee of good quality, but it also has its pitfalls when human behavior is involved and when disagreement occurs between individuals. Quality is assured with a strongly built editorial line and is gained over the years. An academic environment helps to raise quality standards. Many tools are being developed to upraise the quality of Internet products [4]. Some authors argue that it may be impossible to guarantee the quality of medical websites [5].

It is easy to point out that quality is poor on the Internet, but today it can be demonstrated that long-lasting success remains the easiest way to confirm the quality of specialized websites. A specialized website must include all the components of an educational system. To be identified as one of the best educational systems in the world, it must provide a system of worldwide information diffusion with the participation of world-renowned experts. The WebSurg site tries to fulfill these requirements in order to stay at the cutting edge of the virtual education in minimal access surgery. The website is geared to represent the model of the Internet-based virtual university specialized in minimally invasive surgery. The surgical contents are classified into different fields of surgery (e.g., general and digestive, urology, gynecology, endocrine, etc.). A wide range of multimedia technologies helps to maximize presentations of surgical data.

Table 4.1 Results of Google search, 9 March 2005

Keywords	Figures
Training surgery	8,400,000
Education surgery	9,860,000
Laparoscopy surgery	296,000
Laparoscopy education	128,000
Laparoscopy training	116,000

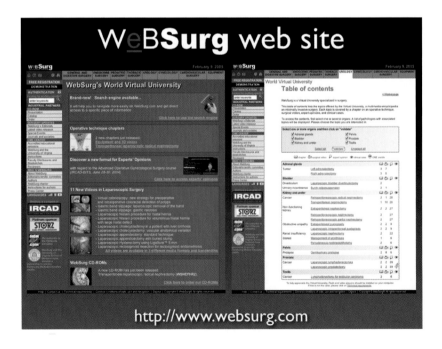

Fig. 4.1 WebSurg website

4.1 Surgical Operative Techniques

The core of the website is made up of surgical operative techniques. One hundred fifty procedures in minimally invasive surgery have been described and posted online. The content of these chapters has been designed for multimedia education and learning. Internationally renowned experts were invited to write texts and send ideas for illustrations. Editors and illustrators worked out an original way of processing such information to provide topnotch illustrations and pictures suitable for visualization on any computer screen. New technologies allow rethinking of the anatomical artwork in order to achieve the best representation from a surgical standpoint. Dedicated software such as Macromedia Flash® technology makes it possible to provide animation to still images. Unlike other media or paper journals, the Internet offers color illustrations, animations, and videos, with no limits in size and number. Internet-based techniques follow the evolution of the technology. Every year a new multimedia version permits to improve the quality of artwork and drawings, to implement new educational tools, as well as to upgrade the existing chapters of operative techniques. The worldwide diffusion of the website mandates an adaptation to the surgeons' culture. For this reason, many chapters are translated into several languages. English, the international language, is complemented with translations into French, and Japanese. At the time of this writing, translation into Chinese was anticipated by the end of 2007. Recently, new software allowed and enhanced

navigation with many functional options including full screen display of information, slide shows, as well as an easy and permanent navigation through the entire chapters of operative techniques with one single mouse click (Fig. 4.2).

4.2 Video Footage

The training of surgeons is continuously making progress with the establishment of structured training standards and criteria to enhance cognitive knowledge by integration of basic science. This has an impact on the clinical and operative skills of surgeons. At present time, videos represent an essential asset of education in minimally invasive surgery, and the rapid evolution of the technology allows high-quality video footage to be made available on the Internet. This possibility will assuredly strongly modify the access to surgical education [6]. The broadcasting of videos through the Internet has been facing technological limits for many years. However, the high-speed Internet broadcasting at present time available (cable and DSL, 512 Kbps and higher) allows the displaying of high-quality, full-screen videos through the Internet. As an example, the WebSurg website gives permanent access to 265 videos of surgical interventions. The evolution of technologies offered Web users the choice of video bandwidth compression for an optimal, high-definition view of the video footage. Each new video published on the website is dis-

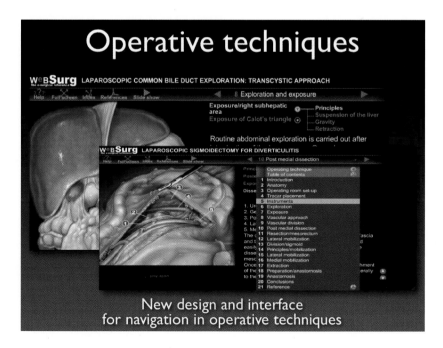

Fig. 4.2 Design of the chapter and interfaces

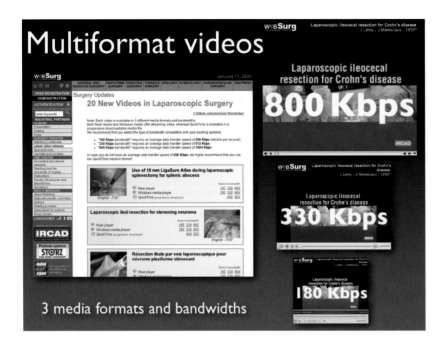

Fig. 4.3 Videos and related bandwidths

played in three bandwidths (180, 330, and 800 Kbps) and in three different player media (Real Player, Windows Media Player, and QuickTime) (Fig. 4.3). The latest videos released on WebSurg are also chronologically sequenced, thereby allowing the surgeon to have direct access to any operative key step in the surgical procedure. The success of these videos is confirmed by the rate of hits on the videos, with an increase of 166% in 2004 (from 14,007 in January to 39,618 in December) (Fig. 4.4). An average visit length of 9 min per connection represents a tremendous achievement for a website dedicated to surgical procedures.

4.3   The Voices and Opinions of the Experts

A teaching tool with the objective of reproducing all aspects of a university school of medicine must incorporate regularly updated information provided by world-renowned experts. To ensure and promote this feature, the website offers more than 500 sequences of experts' opinions, where most recognized experts share their opinion on specific topics in different fields of surgery on a worldwide scale. Experts' opinions represent a huge benefit to any standard teaching tool that would generally present only one specific author's opinion about a given chapter. Multimedia technologies make it possible to simultaneously show and voice various experts' opinions of great expertise in a specific domain of laparoscopic surgery in order to improve the richness and value of the delivered information.

4.4   New Improvements for Access to Surgical Education

Despite the worldwide diffusion of the website http://www.websurg.com, computer access may be considered as restrictive. Computers remain heavy structures and require physical links to provide access to the Internet. Recent developments in wireless access points (WiFi) offer the possibility of getting Internet access without space constraints. On the other hand, most of the professionals manage their schedules and data on personal data assistants (PDAs). Thanks to the latest technological advances, these PDAs allow to display images and sound. The management of data on WebSurg makes it possible to use such technology. Nowadays WebSurg can be connected via PDAs, hence not only increasing its accessibility, but also placing it at the cutting edge of technology.

Giving access to regularly updated data to a greater number of healthcare professionals gives them the possibility of using the latest innovative means of communication.

4.5   Other Educational Services

The educational sector and value of the World Virtual University represented by WebSurg is also complemented by the presentation of typical clinical cases showing outstanding or common data from patients operated on by laparoscopy.

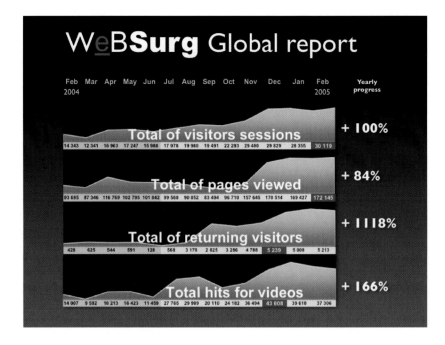

Fig. 4.4 WebSurg's report connections: hits, visitors, videos

Validation of knowledge is more and more under the supervision of governments with their own requirements of nationally approved CME for physicians in order to maintain medical licensure. In the United States, the accreditation of CME activities is provided by the Accreditation Council for Continuing Medical Education (ACCME) [7]. Today the Internet represents one of the typical means of obtaining CME. With the geometric expansion of information exchange via the Internet, online CME activities have become a new, inexpensive, and convenient way of obtaining CME credit hours. According to the 2003 Annual Report from the ACCME, 8,376 CME activities were obtained (275 were available online, for a total 34,535 credit hours). These opportunities were characterized as both live online webcast and/or enduring materials, directly or jointly sponsored.

At present, the WebSurg website offers 24 hours of category 1 credit through different accredited educational sessions with the partnership of the University of Mc Master University (Canada). In 2004, 467 website members validated a number of 1,120 CME credit hours. The WebSurg chapters comply with the requirements of the ACCME, since they are structured like a self-containing learning program that can be viewed independently. Self-assessment questions in the form of a posttest follow each learning session and provide the validation of major concepts in the learning activity.

Web-based learning is considered an effective, well-accepted, and efficient means of educating physicians [8]. It allows for fast access to information, which has never been realized before. However, the credibility and reliability of this information remains a factor that the physician must confirm while obtaining this information on the Web. Furthermore, many of the Web evaluation systems commonly evaluate a website, not just a webpage. For example, a website may fulfill all the requirements for an acceptable site, but then only offer various degrees in the quality of information given. Therefore, with the current Web evaluation systems, a verification of the whole site is not possible, nor is the attribution of a guarantee of quality to the whole site possible. Because of this, CME chapters must be validated one after the other for their entire content, which has sometimes to be partially rewritten or re-edited to reflect the standard practice but not the innovative technique. Therefore, an entire website cannot be validated for CME globally.

In the evaluation of websites, the number of active members and pages viewed are not as important as the total number of returning visitors. The number of registered members and pages viewed cannot be considered the major indicator of guaranteeing quality for any website. The total number of returning visitors may appear to be a good token of satisfaction concerning the quality of the scientific surgical content provided. As an example, the website, www.websurg.com has over 35,000 registered members and 17,474 active members who get connected to the website more than one time in a 12-month time span. In our example, the number of returning visitors has increased 1,118% on a monthly basis, from 428 in January 2004 to more than 5,000 in December 2004 (Fig. 4.4). This is apparently related to the diffusion of regularly renewed live videos of surgical procedures. This high rate of return of visitors means that surgeons, when looking for a specific piece of information on the website, consider the content of the site as credible and reliable, allowing them to return on the website for further information.

The sense of quality is also correlated with the Internet connectivity and access speed dependent on the technology used for hosting and streaming of information. WebSurg has chosen a high-quality professional hosting center. France Telecom technology offers dedicated servers, allowing high-speed connection as well as security and firewall systems. This has been made available thanks to redundant server, load balancer, and a support service working 24 hours a day. The content delivery network is ensured by the Akamai Platform, allowing the streamlining and broadcasting of videos and operative technique chapters all over the world through 14,000 servers located in 65 countries.

The global quality of the website is also reinforced as all partners, contributors, and users are in agreement.

The factors that may compromise the reputation of an information media source were listed by Davis et al. [9]:

- Publishing material not subjected to a rigorous peer review process
- Apparent favoritism towards specific authors, institutions, or even topics
- Strategic placement or advertisement next to relevant articles
- Frequent publication of symposia or of single products
- Product placement in report on supposedly independent studies
- Promotion of sectarian interest disguised as independent commentary
- Failure to disclose conflict of interest

"Transgression in any of these areas leads to a rapid diminution of trust in the journal's standards and thus a falling reputation, a downwards spiral to mediocrity and scientific marginalization" [9]. Therefore, editors and authors must acquire and comply with the constraints of reading on the Internet. The way of presenting information has to be adapted, the text shortened, and the imagination stimulated for a new way of illustration. The peer review process must also be adapted to this type of format. The most original part of WebSurg's Virtual University is the possibility of adding videos of experts' opinions in a form of peer review. Therefore, reviewers do not influence the content, but have the possibility to add further information in order to moderate the conclusions made by the authors. In fact, the functions of a website owner and editors of that site must be different in order to avoid any con-

flict of interest. Advertisement has to be separated from the scientific content. This aspect pinpoints the issue of the funding of websites. Educational websites are not to be compared to the "business-to-consumer" model. Independent institutions have to establish a clear partnership with industries, universities, and government institutions to have the possibility of keeping their independence in the development of the website. The Internet represents an entirely new media with an unlimited potential to create, manage, and distribute knowledge. With this in mind, the re-engineering of the knowledge base of a standard university led to the concept of World Virtual University as a service institution for surgeons. Typically, a single institution cannot provide all the data for education in any topic. The Virtual University Institution structures and categorizes knowledge by managing the data available. The role of the Virtual University is to diffuse this knowledge to its participants in the most efficient manner possible.

WebSurg, with approximately 30,000 monthly visitors' sessions, represents an original contribution to what is now referred to as multimedia e-learning and e-training by using the latest technologies to display videos, texts, and illustrations simultaneously. To achieve such goals, it must be noted that the extraordinary influence of WebSurg is the result of significantly great effort put into the project by professionals as well as significant costs. In fact, the development of www.websurg.com has required a financial investment of $20 million over a 5-year period, involving over 45 full-time salaried employees. The success can only be the result of professional self-commitment and positive attitude.

The dramatic worldwide increase in bandwidths helps to increase the speed of this information, as it is displayed and stored all over the world. It will certainly help in the development of nations that had, until recently, under-equipped transmission systems, such as China or India. It is countries and cultures such as these that now represent the future economic power of the world due to their size as these two countries alone represent a third of the worldwide population. The very nature of the Virtual University, with its multilingual abilities, follows this and other growing trends to educate the surgeons of today and the future.

References

1. Butler D (2005) Publishers irritated by Google's digital library. Nature 433:446
2. Dutson E, Maisonneuve H, Bouabene A, Leroy J, Chekan E (2003) Is the Internet a viable method to obtain surgical continuing medical Education? Surg Endosc 17:S249

3. Gandsas A, Draper K, Chekan E, Garcia-Oria M, McMahon RL, Clary EM, Monnig R, Eubanks S (2001) Laparoscopy and the Internet: a surgeon survey. Surg Endosc 15:1044–1048

4. Eysenbach G, Diepgen TL (1998) Towards quality management of medical information on the Internet: evaluation, labelling and filtering the information. Br Med J 317:1496–1502

5. Delamothe T (2000) Quality of websites: kite marking the west wind. Rating the quality of medical websites may be impossible. Br Med J 321:843–844

6. Ellis DG, Mayrose J (2003) The success of emergency telemedicine at the State University of New York at Buffalo. Telemed J E Health 9:73–79

7. Accreditation Council for Continuing Medical Education (2003) ACCME annual report data. http://www.accme.org. Accessed 15 March 2005

8. Cook DA, Dupras DM, Thompson WG, Pankratz VS (2005) Web-based learning in residents' continuity clinics: a randomized, controlled trial. Acad Med 80:90–97

9. Davies HTO, Rennie D (1999) Independence, governance, and trust. Redefining the relationship between JAMA and the AMA. JAMA 281:2344–2346

Virtual Reality: Objective Assessment, Education, and Training

5

Anthony G. Gallagher, E. Matt Ritter

Computer-based simulation has been used for decades in aviation and other professional fields. However, the last 15 years have seen numerous attempts to introduce computer-based simulation into clinical medicine. Surgery, and specifically minimally invasive surgery (MIS), has led the way in the development and application of this technology in clinical practice. Recently, use of computer-based simulation for training has expanded into the multidisciplinary fields of catheter-based, image-guided intervention, enabling both surgeons and non-surgeons alike to train on new procedures. The widespread introduction and use of computer-based simulation is changing the way physicians are trained and positively affecting the treatments patients receive. We believe that this revolution represents a paradigm shift in the way procedural-based medicine will be learned and practiced.

The terms *virtual reality* and *computer-based simulation* are often used interchangeably. Virtual reality, or VR, commonly refers to "a computer-generated representation of an environment that allows sensory interaction, thus giving the impression of actually being present" [1]. However, VR is probably best defined by Riva [2], who suggested that it was a communication interface based on interactive visualization that allows the user to interface, interact with, and integrate different types of sensory inputs that simulate important aspects of real world experience. It allows the user to interact and experience important aspects of the encounter rather than simply observing. This interaction has important learning implications, which is highlighted shortly. Although first proposed as a training strategy for surgery in 1991 by Satava [3], acceptance of the use of VR for training approach has been slow due to costs, skepticism within the medical community, and the lack robust scientific evidence to support the efficacy and effectiveness of this training strategy. However, this is rapidly changing.

The first VR surgical simulator in laparoscopic surgery was designed by Satava (1993) [3]. He developed it primarily as a training tool to help counteract many of the difficulties he observed many of his colleagues were having in acquiring the skills for endoscopic surgery. However, because of the limitations in computer processing capacity, the virtual abdomen was cartoon-like in appearance. Despite this, the simulation was realistic in its anatomical and technical accuracy, allowing trainees the ability to practice skills outside the operating theater in a computer-based environment.

There have been numerous developments in VR simulators since 1991, and these have been reviewed elsewhere [4]. However, we believe that more can be learned from an in-depth analysis of our experience of one particular simulator, the Minimally Invasive Surgical Trainer – Virtual Reality (MIST-VR), over the last decade. Although this represents the experience on a single simulator that trains and assesses simple surgical skills, the principles are applicable to all types of simulators.

One of the things that our experience with this simulator has taught us is that most surgeons are very naive when evaluating the functionality of simulators. Surgeons tend to evaluate simulators on a very superficial level, i.e., does it look like "real surgery," rather than how the instruments or tissue behave, how appropriate the metrics are, or most importantly how appropriate is the simulation curriculum. In the past, surgeons believed that there were two important requisites of any surgical simulator, an accurate depiction of detail and a high level of interactivity. Many felt that organs must be anatomically correct and have appropriate natural properties when grasped, clamped, or cut. Many surgeons believed that grasping an object without weight, shape, or texture made training in a virtual environment insubstantial. However, the best validated VR simulator in medicine, the MIST-VR, has demonstrated these beliefs to be at least partly incorrect.

Another important advantage of computer-based (including VR) simulators is that objective criteria must be built into the simulator to support the assessment tools. The student then trains until they reach the criterion, at which time they are said to have achieved a proficiency level. The proficiency level is established by having an experienced (expert) surgeon perform on the simulator until the surgeon's learning curve is flat for two consecutive trials (frequently by the third or fourth trial). These values then define the benchmark criteria, the figure of merit to which the student must achieve before going to the next task or until completing training on the simulator and graduating to the operating room.

5.1   Simulation Development: Lessons Learned

The first important lesson to be learned about the MIST-VR is that it was developed by a collaborative group including an engineer (Chris Sutton, London), the end user, i.e., a surgeon (Dr. Rory McCloy, Manchester), and an expert in curriculum/metrics development, i.e., a psychologist (Dr. Bob Stone, Manchester). Many simulators are developed by an engineer who has consulted an end user rather than intimately involving them, and rarely are a curriculum development and metrics expert involved. Much like a scientific experiment, a simulator is much more difficult to fix at the end of development than at the beginning. For optimal development, these groups need to be intimately involved at the outset. The experts must also be cognizant of the cost implications of their suggestions weighed against what it truly adds to the simulation. Lastly, in the development of a simulator, surgeons must give very serious consideration to the fidelity, i.e., anatomical realism, haptic feedback, and metrics, they require for the accruement of clinical benefit. One common mistake is that the simulation must look ultrarealistic. In many circumstances, especially when dealing with basic skills and novices, it is preferable to have a lower-fidelity graphic representation that accurately trains and assesses simple skills. Of paramount importance is to perform a task deconstruction (divide the task into its simplest components) and task analysis to ensure that the skills (hand motions, etc.) are correctly presented to the student in the simplest manner. Once simple tasks are mastered, then more complex, higher resolution simulations can be performed.

Our experience with the MIST-VR bears directly on this point. The MIST-VR system was designed to develop and assess minimally invasive surgical skills, using advanced computer technology in a format that could be easily operated by both tutor and trainee. The system is composed of a frame equipped with two standard laparoscopic instruments. This hardware is interfaced with a PC running the MIST-VR software. The software creates a virtual environment on the display screen and is able to track and display the position and movement of the instruments in real time. An accurately scaled operating volume of 10 cm³ is represented by a three-dimensional cube on the computer screen. The overall image size and the sizes of the target object can be varied for different skill levels. Targets appear randomly within the operating volume according to the task and can be "grasped" and "manipulated" [5].

In training mode, the program guides the trainee through a series of six tasks that progressively become more complex, enabling the development of hand–eye motor coordination essential for the safe clinical practice of laparoscopic surgery. Each task is based on an essential surgical technique employed in MIS (see above). Performance is scored for time, error rate, and efficiency of movement for each task, for both hands. Every time a trainee logs onto the system a record of the trainee's performance is stored in a database, thus providing an objective record of the trainee's progress. The ability to review the database can help the trainer identify specific areas for further practice. Together these features of the MIST-VR may help to establish objective standards of accomplishment and help to identify when a trainee is ready to enter the operating theatre. In achieving the proficiency level to graduate to the operating room, the MIST-VR can be practiced as often as the student chooses, reviewing the student's performance after each trial, and without requiring the presence of a faculty or observer—the system automatically assesses and reports the performance to the student. With little time for faculty to devote to training, this aspect of simulators is of great value.

5.2   Simulation Training: Evidence-Based Adoption?

In 1997 both Prof. Sir Ara Darzi's group at St. Mary's, London, and Dr. Tony Gallagher's group working at Queen's University, Belfast, were asked by a large US laparoscopic instrument manufacturer to conduct a preliminary evaluation of the MIST-VR [6, 7]. Preliminary results from both groups were positive. Despite these encouraging results, the initial response of the international laparoscopic surgical community was the MIST-VR simply did not look or feel like laparoscopic surgery. As a follow-up to this preliminary work, an extensive list of scientifically robust studies demonstrating that when training with the MIST-VR was objectively compared to the current standard of training for the development of laparoscopic skills, the MIST-VR produced skills that were at least as good as, or good but usually better than, the conventional training program. Despite these studies the surgical community remained unconvinced. Many skeptics pointed to the fact that all of these initial studies simply demonstrated that training on the simulator improved performance on tasks in the skills laboratory and did not demonstrate benefits in operative performance. This was a valid criticism which needed to be addressed. In 2001, a multidisciplinary team at Yale University conducted a prospective, randomized, double-blind clinical trial to test whether training on the MIST-VR translated into improved intraoperative performance. The trial compared the performance of a group of residents who received standard surgical residency training to a matched group who received proficiency-based training on the MIST-VR; that is, the residents trained as many trials as necessary to reach the criteria and achieve the proficiency level. Both groups then were objectively assessed on their ability to dissect the gallbladder from the liver bed during a laparoscopic cholecystectomy [8].

The results of this study showed training on the simulator significantly improved intraoperative performance. VR trained residents performed the procedure 30% faster and made six times fewer objectively assessed intraoperative errors when compared with the standard-trained residents. Although the number of subjects was small ($n = 16$), the statistical power of this effect was 0.9996. These results have been independently replicated in Denmark [9].

The response of the surgical community to the results of this study was mixed; for some this was enough to convince them that simulation was a powerful training tool. However, the majority clung to the criticism that while the study was well designed, the small number of subjects and the fact that only part of the procedure had been performed reduced its widespread acceptance. In October 2004 at the [10] Clinical Congress of the American College of Surgeons, another prospective, randomized, double-blind trial from Emory University was reported, which used the exact same experimental design as the Yale study. However, there were two important differences: in the Emory study subject's performance was assessed on the full laparoscopic cholecystectomy procedure, and the Emory study used only surgical residents in postgraduate years 1 and 2, whereas the Yale study used residents in years 1–4. Again, the VR-trained group significantly outperformed the standard trained groups. We believe these results demonstrate two very powerful things, the first being that simulation, when applied correctly to training, succeeds in improving performance, and the second is that even a low-fidelity VR simulator such as the MIST-VR can produce a very powerful training effect. Why does simulation training produce such a powerful training effect? The answers lie in the understanding of the importance of metrics and application of simulation adhering to sound principles of education and training.

5.3 Metrics for Objective Assessment

Computer-based simulation has several advantages when compared with conventional methods for surgical training. One of the major advantages of computer-based simulation is that the same experience or sequence of events can be replicated repeatedly. This repetition allows the trainee to learn from mistakes in a safe environment. Another benefit that is probably equally if not more important is the objective feedback a trainee can receive from a computer-based simulator. Since everything a trainee "does" on a computer-based simulator is essentially data, all actions can be tracked by the computer. In addition to crude measures such as performance time, detailed data such as instrument path length, speed of instrument movement, and the exact location in space of any instrument at any point in time is recorded. While this data alone is meaningless, it can be used by subject matter experts to create a set of very robust and objective performance metrics. A simulator without metrics is really no better than an expensive video game. While the main function of metrics is to provide the trainee with objective and proximate feedback on performance, they also allow the trainer to objectively assess the progress of the trainee throughout the training process. This allows the trainer to provide formative feedback to aid the trainee in acquiring skill. While providing this formative feedback is currently the most valuable function of objective assessment with simulation, inevitably simulators will be used for summative performance assessment. This testing will then be used for processes such as selection and credentialing in the future, much like knowledge testing is used now. In order for simulators to be applied to such high-stakes assessment, a much more rigorous set of metrics is required, and is still in the experimental phase. When this does come to the fore it is certain the metrics for that simulator must be shown meet the same psychometric standards of validation as any other psychometric test [15].

The formulation of metrics requires breaking down a task into its essential components (see above: task deconstruction, task analysis) and then tightly defining what differentiates optimal from suboptimal performance. Unfortunately this aspect of simulation has been given all too little attention by the simulation industry. Drawing on the example from the MIS community, almost all of the VR simulators use execution time as a metric. Unfortunately time analyzed as an independent variable is at best crude and at worst a dangerous metric. If one thinks of performance as being a function of time and quality, the relationship can be represented by the following equation:

$$\text{Performance} \sim \frac{\text{Quality}}{\text{Time}}$$

Thus, performance is directly proportional to quality and inversely proportional to time. With this relationship, if quality is held constant and time decreases, then performance is improved. Conversely if a large increase in quality is gained from a minimal increase in time, performance is still improved despite the longer execution time. While this is obviously an oversimplified relationship, it serves to illustrate the importance of the fact that if time is to be used as a metric, some metrics to assess quality must also be included.

For example, in the MIS environment, being able to tie an intracorporeal knot quickly gives no indication of the quality of the knot. A poorly tied knot can obviously lead to a multitude of complications. There are only a few reports in the literature that use objective quality analysis because of the difficulty in acquiring this type of information, but this type of information is greatly facilitated in the computer-based environment.

There is no magic solution to the issue of quality metrics, and it is almost certain that good metrics will have to be simulator and procedure specific. For example, as we have illustrated, while time alone is not a crucial metric for MIS procedure performance, time and the resultant radiation exposure is very critical in the assessment of performance in many image-guided, catheter-based procedures where extreme doses of radiation can lead to burns and other dire consequences.

Quality measures can be assessed both inside and outside of the computer-aided environment. The Imperial College laparoscopic group, led by Sir Ara Darzi, has been researching economy of hand movement for number of years by an electromagnetic tracking system they have developed (ICSAD) [11]. What they have found is that experienced surgeons have a smoother instrument path trajectory in comparison with less experienced surgeons. The elegance of this approach is that the system can be used to assess open as well as MIS skills. Other groups [12–14] have been using different metrics such as performance variability and errors as a key indicator of skill level. Senior or experienced surgeons perform well and consistently—the reduction of variability is an extremely important aspect of a proficient surgeon, so training to be consistent is as important as training to be proficient.

The most valuable metrics that a simulation can provide is identification of errors. The whole point of training is to improve performance, make performance consistent, and reduce errors. Simulation designers must take great care to create error metrics that both train safe behavior as well as not allow unsafe behavior. As mentioned previously, one of the major benefits of simulation is that trainees are allowed to make mistakes in a consequence-free environment, before they ever perform that procedure on a patient. But if a simulator allows a trainee to perform an unsafe maneuver without identifying it as an error, dangerous behaviors can be trained, possibly becoming difficult to untrain later. Thus, omitting important error metrics and allowing unsafe behavior must be avoided, and this requires close collaboration with procedure content experts who are also familiar with simulation. The end result of a good simulator with well-designed metrics is a training system where trainees can learn both what *to* do and what *not* to do when operating on patients. In the didactic part of the curriculum, the student must be taught exactly what the error is, and then should be tested (written) to ensure that the student is able to identify when he or she make an error, before starting on the simulator. The errors must be quantified so as to be completely unambiguous. Without robust metrics the simulator is at best an expensive video game, and at worst an adverse outcome waiting to happen.

5.4 Education and Training

The current published evidence clearly demonstrates that VR simulation can improve intraoperative performance. There seems to be some confusion as to whether simulators *educate* or *train* individuals, and the two terms are often used interchangeably. Simulation is frequently referred to as education rather than training, or education and training. Although closely related, education and training are not the same. Education usually refers to the communication or acquisition of knowledge or information, whereas training refers to the acquisition of skills (cognitive or psychomotor). Individuals being prepared to perform a procedure need to know what *to* do, what *not* to do, how to do what they need to do, and how to identify when they have made mistakes. Most available VR simulators provide technical skills training. They primarily teach the trainee *how* to perform the procedure and do not concentrate on the didactic information that the physician should know to efficiently and safely deal with adverse events such as complications or unusual anatomy. This however is not always the case.

A VR-based training study for carotid angiography in which preliminary results were reported at Medicine Meets Virtual Reality 2005, lends support to the power of VR simulation as both an education and a training tool. This study compares in vivo hands-on–mentored catheterization training in comparison with VR-based training for carotid angiography. The subjects are senior attending interventional cardiologist and fellows. Preliminary results are very compelling in favor of the VR-trained group in terms of catheter and wire-handling skills; based on the results of other simulators, this outcome is what was expected. However, one of the preliminary findings that we were not expecting is that the VR-trained group outperformed the standard training group with respect to acquiring the appropriate cranial and vasculature fluoroscopic images during the assessment procedure. This is not really a technical skill but rather knowledge-based skill. On considering this finding, the most reasonable explanation is that the VR trainees were acquiring knowledge about important aspects of the procedure such as order and image orientation while they were as a priority acquiring the technical skills. So while the benefit of VR as a training tool has been well demonstrated, its power as an educational tool may currently be underestimated.

5.5 Simulation Fidelity: Are Graphics Enough?

While one of the advantages of training on a high-fidelity, full-procedural simulator may be additional knowledge accrual, this should not be interpreted as a mandate that all types of computer-based simulation must be high-fidelity. In reality, there are many other means of conveying this knowledge-based information that will be equally or more effective with considerably less cost. The main function of a simulator is, in fact, that the cognitive component of technical skills training should be acquired prior to the psychomotor skills training on the simulator. As simulator fidelity increases so does the price of some current high-fidelity simulators, costing anywhere from $100,000 to over $1 million. Thus end users of surgical simulation must assess how much fidelity is required to achieve the greatest return on investment. The data from the MIST-VR clinical trials clearly demonstrate that a low-fidelity simulator can consistently improve intraoperative performance. However, this does not mean that simulation fidelity is unimportant. Consider, a straightforward laparoscopic cholecystectomy performed by a surgical resident under the direct guidance of an attending/consultant surgeon in the operating room. This is not a particularly high-risk training situation, and the risk of a life-threatening or life-altering complication is very low [16]. Conversely, an endovascular surgeon performing a carotid angioplasty and stenting procedure carries much more risk. Results from the only multispecialty prospective randomized trial on this procedure performed by experienced physicians showed that the risk of stroke or death at 30 days was as high as 4.6% [17]. In a high-risk procedure such as carotid angioplasty and stenting, the fidelity of the simulator should be maximized in attempt to replicate the exact procedure as closely as possible to take every step possible to minimize patient risk.

Another important point to make about fidelity of a simulator is that fidelity goes beyond computer graphics and presentation. Unfortunately many surgeons are overawed by and place too much emphasis on the pure graphics aspect of the simulator. In a high-fidelity simulation, the tissue and instruments should behave as close as possible to how they would in a patient. The instruments must not behave as if there is a predefined path for them or automatically tie the knot, and tissue

behavior should also be as realistic as possible. A high-fidelity simulator must allow the trainee to make mistakes (both cognitive and psychomotor skills) and learn from these mistakes and the trainee's performance must be meaningfully quantified, with well–thought out metrics that distinguish between those who are good at the procedure and those who are not. A robust but very simple toolkit of reports for the analysis of performance should be incorporated into the simulator to give clear and easily understood feedback when an error is made. If surgeons ignore or fail to appreciate this issue, we risk spending large amounts of resources for simulators that will not meet our needs.

5.6 Simulation as Part of the Curriculum

Whether a high-fidelity, full-procedural or low-fidelity, basic training simulator is purchased, it should be remembered that it is only a tool that must be integrated into a well-developed curriculum to be effective. Inappropriate application of simulation will lead the user to the erroneous belief that simulation does not work. So how should simulators be appropriately applied to a training curriculum? The goal of current simulation-based training is to create a pretrained novice. This term describes an individual who may have little or no experience with performing the actual procedure, but who has trained to the point where many of the required fundamental skills have already been mastered. With this accomplished, the trainee can devote nearly all of his or her attentional resources to learning the details of performing the actual procedure, such as how to identify the correct dissection planes or how to gain exposure in the operative field instead of concentrating on what his or her hands are doing. This results in optimization of the operating room experience, reduces frustration of both the trainee and mentor, and it should result in accelerated learning.

To achieve this goal, a training curriculum must be structured to optimize the skills gained from the simulator. Any valid simulator will have the ability to distinguish between the performance of individuals who are already proficient at the skill being trained, and those who are not. Using the carefully developed metrics and setting the criteria by which the figure of merit for the proficiency level is determined as discussed previously, the simulator can then objectively assess and quantify the performance of the proficient individual. This objectively determined proficiency level can then be used as a goal for those training on the simulator and in fact, this is the key aspect of implementing a successful simulation training curriculum. Training on the simulator should not be complete until the trainee has reached an objectively established level of proficiency.

As a guide to curriculum development, the design of any curriculum should contain 6 sequential parts: (1) anatomy instruction, (2) steps of the procedure, (3) identification of errors, (4) a written test to insure cognitive knowledge, (5) skills training and assessment on the simulator, and (6) results reporting and feedback to student.

5.7   Training to Proficiency on a VR Simulator

The traditional way that simulation has been applied to training is through a prescriptive approach. Typically the trainee is required to train for a prespecified number of trials or number of hours. However, all that this approach achieves is considerable variability in posttraining skills [18]. Individuals start from different baseline skill levels, they learn at different rates, and some are more gifted than others. Simulation allows for leveling of the playing field and sets a skill benchmark, which as individual can reach at his or her own pace. Individuals should also not be allowed to progress to the next phase of training until they demonstrate they are performing proficiently and consistently. When setting the proficiency level, the surgeons used to set the standard do not need to be the best of the best; rather, they should reflect a representative sample of the proficient population. If the proficiency level is set too high, trainees will never reach it and if set too low, an inferior skills set will be produced. Ideally, proficiency levels should be set nationally or internationally. While national or international proficiency levels on VR simulators may be some way off, proficiency levels can be set locally in each training program or hospital. The Yale VR to OR study and the Emory VR to OR study has shown the power of this approach [8, 10]. The whole point of training is not simply to improve performance, but also to make it more consistent. Indeed performing well consistently is emerging as one of the key indicators of training success [8, 12].

Proficiency-based training as a new approach to the acquisition of procedural-based medical skills took a giant leap forward in April 2004. As part of the roll-out of a new device for carotid angioplasty and stenting, the US Food and Drug Administration (FDA) mandated, as part of the device approval package, metric-based training to proficiency on a VR simulator as the required training approach for physicians who will be using the new device [19]. The company manufacturing the carotid stent system informed the FDA that they would educate physicians with a tiered training approach utilizing an online, multimedia, didactic package, and training of catheter and wire-handling skills with a high-fidelity VR simulator, using a curriculum based on achieving a level of proficiency in both the didactic and technical areas. What this approach allows is for training of physicians who enter training with variable knowledge, skill, and experience, but leave with objectively assessed proficient knowledge and skills. This is particularly important for a procedure like carotid angioplasty and stenting, as it crosses multiple clinical specialties with each bringing a different skill set to the training table. For example, a vascular surgeon has a thorough cognitive understanding of vascular anatomy and management of carotid disease, but may lack some of the psychomotor technical skills of wire and catheter manipulation. Conversely, an interventional cardiologist may have all of the technical skill, but may not be as familiar with the anatomical and clinical management issues. A sound training strategy must ensure that all of these specialists are able to meet an objectively assessable minimum level of proficiency in all facets of the procedure. We believe that this development represents a paradigm shift in the way procedural-based medicine is trained and will result in a reduction in turf wars concerning future credentialing for new procedures. As long as a physician is able to demonstrate that he or she possesses the requisite knowledge and skills to perform a procedure, specialty affiliation will become irrelevant. Overall, we see this development as a good thing for surgery, procedural-based medicine, and for patient safety.

5.8   Conclusion

Computer-based simulation or VR simulation in surgery has been around for more than a decade and a half, but has only recently begun to gain momentum. Despite considerable early skepticism, there is now a growing body of level 1 objective evidence to show that properly applied computer-based simulation training strategies can improve performance of surgical trainees. Developing simulators to produce these results is not easy and must be done collaboratively with experts in computer science, engineering, medicine, and behavioral and educational science to produce a robust training tool. Graphics and good looks are not enough, and robust metrics must be in place to help trainees learn both what *to* and what *not* to do. Finally, simulation must be incorporated as a piece of an overall education and training curriculum designed to produce a pre-trained novice with consistently reproducible skills.

Ironically, a training solution [20] that was proposed more than a decade and a half ago to help solve skills problems in laparoscopic surgery is helping to change the training paradigm in all of procedural based medicine. It is an approach to training that his here to stay.

References

1. Coleman J, Nduka CC, Darzi A (1994) Virtual reality and laparoscopic surgery. Brit J Surg 8:1709–1711
2. Riva G (2003) Applications of virtual environments in medicine. Methods Inf Med 42:524–534
3. Satava RM (1993) Virtual reality surgical simulator: the first steps. Surg Endosc 7:203–205
4. Schijven M, Jakimowicz J (2003) Virtual reality surgical laparoscopic simulators. Surg Endosc 12:1943–1950
5. Wilson MS, Middlebrook A, Sutton C, Stone R, McCloy RF (1997) MISTVR: a virtual reality trainer for laparoscopic surgery assesses performance. Ann R Coll Surg 79:403–404
6. Taffinder N, Sutton C, Fishwick RJ, McManus IC, Darzi A (1998) Validation of virtual reality to teach and assess psychomotor skills in laparoscopic surgery: results from randomised controlled studies using the MISTVR laparoscopic simulator. In: Westwood JD, Hoffman HM, Stredney D, Weghorst SJ (eds) Medicine meets virtual reality. IOS/Ohmsha, Amsterdam
7. Gallagher AG, McClure N, McGuigan J, Crothers I, Browning J (1999) Virtual reality training in laparoscopic surgery: a preliminary assessment of Minimally Invasive Surgical Trainer Virtual Reality (MIST-VR). Endoscopy 31:310–313
8. Seymour N, Gallagher A, Roman S et al (2002) Virtual reality training improves operating room performance: results of a randomized, double-blinded study. Ann of Surg 236:458–464
9. Grantcharov TP, Kristianson VB, Bendix J, Bardram L, Rosenerg J, Funch-Jensen P (2004) Randomized clinical trial of virtual reality simulation for laparoscopic skills training. Br J Surg 91:146–150
10. McClusky DA, Gallagher AG, Ritter EM, Lederman AB, Van Sickle KR, Baghai M, Smith CD (2004) Virtual reality training improves junior residents' operating room performance: results of a prospective randomized double-blinded study of the complete laparoscopic cholecystectomy. J Am Coll Surg 199(Suppl):3
11. Datta V, Mackay S, Mandalia M, Darzi A (2001) The use of electromagnetic motion tracking analysis to objectively measure open surgical skill in the laboratory-based model. J Am Coll Surg 193:479–185
12. Gallagher AG, Satava RM (2002) Objective assessment of experience, junior and novice laparoscopic performance with virtual reality: learning curves and reliability measures. Surg Endosc 16:1746–1752
13. Ritter E, McClusky D, Gallagher A et al (2003) Objective psychomotor skills assessment of experienced and novice flexible endoscopists with a virtual reality simulator. J Gastrointest Surg 7:871–878
14. Tang B, Hanna GB, Joice P, Cuschieri A (2004) Identification and categorization of technical errors by Observational Clinical Human Reliability Assessment (OCHRA) during laparoscopic cholecystectomy. Arch Surg 139:1215–1220
15. Gallagher AG, Ritter EM, Satava RM (2003) Fundamental principles of validation, and reliability: rigorous science for the assessment of surgical education and training. Surg Endosc 10:1525–1529
16. Denziel D, Millikan KW, Economou SG, Doolas A, Ko ST, Airan MC (1993) Complications of laparoscopic cholecystectomy: a national survey of 4,292 hospitals and an analysis of 77,604 cases. Am J Surg 165:9–14
17. Yadav JS, Wholey MH, Kuntz RE, Fayad P, Katzen BT, Mishkel GJ, Bajwa TK, Whitlow P, Strickman NE, Jaff MR, Popma JJ, Snead DB, Cutlip DE, Firth BG, Ouriel K (2004) Stenting and angioplasty with protection in patients at high risk for endarterectomy investigators. Protected carotid-artery stenting versus endarterectomy in high-risk patients. N Engl J Med 351:1493–1501
18. Gallagher AG, Ritter EM, Champion H, Higgins G, Fried MP, Moses G, Smith CD, Satava RM (2005) Virtual reality simulation for the operating room: proficiency-based training as a paradigm shift in surgical skills training. Ann Surg 241:364–372
19. Gallagher AG, Cates CU (2004) Approval of virtual reality training for carotid stenting: what this means for procedural-based medicine. JAMA 292:3024–302626
20. Satava RM (1996) Advanced simulation technologies for surgical education. Bull Am Coll Surg 81:77–81

Organizing Surgical Simulation Centers in Response to Disruptive Technologies

Mark W. Bowyer*

Medical knowledge continues to expand rapidly, and surgeons are faced with increasing numbers of surgical procedures that must be learned and mastered. This revolution is occurring against a backdrop in which practitioners are required to become more efficient in patient care, with fewer hours available for teaching and learning. The added pressure of reduced work hours has led to limited options for responding to new disruptive technologies. When a new procedure such as laparoscopic cholecystectomy is introduced, how can large numbers of practicing surgeons and residents in training be trained to be safe and efficient without compromising patient care? The American College of Surgeons (ACS) has recognized this problem and has formulated an ad hoc committee to create a model for what will ultimately be ACS-approved regional skills centers that will offer surgeons, surgical residents, and medical students opportunities to acquire and maintain surgical skills, as well as learn new procedures and the use of emerging technologies.

Thomas Russell, the current executive director of the ACS, stated "The competitive surgeon of the next 10 to 20 years will need to possess a different set of skills than we have needed in the past" [1]. Dr. Russell has suggested that the use of simulation will provide early exposure to medical students, piquing their interest in a surgical career. Resident education will involve the use of simulators and experiences outside the operating room (OR) to enhance the core competencies and move the learning process away from the traditional approach of "see one, do one, teach one" to "see one, practice many, and do one" [1]. The surgeon of the future will be required to have periodic cognitive testing every few years as well as testing of their technological skills with the use of simulators as they progress in their careers. The acquisition of new surgical skills in practice will be much more structured in the future. The practice of industry-sponsored short courses with rapid introduction into clinical practice will no longer be acceptable. Surgeons will likely be required to undergo retraining in regional centers in which skills can be learned through validated multimodality curriculum.

A prime example of this is the carotid stenting procedure, which was recently approved by the US Food and Drug Administration (FDA). The new twist to this is that the FDA (for the first time) has mandated that all practitioners must train "to proficiency" on a simulator before they can perform the procedure on humans [2].

There is clearly an obvious need to develop skills centers to respond to the educational needs of new and potentially disruptive technologies. This chapter makes the case for the use of simulation to meet the educational needs of surgeons in the future, with a brief overview of the current state of simulation and simulators. In addition, a view of how centers should be organized in the future to meet these needs will be proposed, using an existing facility, the National Capital Area Medical Simulation Center, as an example of one institutions attempt to meet the challenge of responding to disruptive technologies.

6.1 Making the Case for Simulation for Medical Education

In 2000, the Institute of Medicine released its report "To Err is Human: Building a Safer Health System" [3]. This study noted that at least 44,000 Americans die from medical errors every year. As part of the plan for improvement, the authors stated in their recommendations that health care organizations should incorporate proven methods of training such as simulation. Though it may be too early to conclude that simulation in general is a "proven" method, this report certainly has placed the onus on the medical community to challenge the traditional medical education approach and address methods for reducing medical error.

The traditional surgical training method of see one, do one, teach one, in and out of the OR has recently undergone reappraisal. Studies have shown that for a variety of diagnostic and therapeutic procedures, clinicians doing this first few to several dozen cases are more likely to make a greater number of errors (the learning

* The opinions or assertions contained herein are the private views of the authors and are not to be construed as official, or as reflecting the views of the Department of the Army, Department of the Navy, the Advanced Research Projects Agency, or the Department of Defense.

curve) [4]. Some might argue that it has become unreasonable that patients be victims of medical invasive procedural training. On-the-job training with patients can result in prolonged invasive procedures, a potential for erroneous diagnoses, increased patient discomfort, and increased risk for procedure-related morbidity [5].

In many ways, the OR is a poor classroom for learning surgical skills. By necessity, there are several distractions, most having nothing to do with education, that take priority (patient issues) [6]. In general, the opportunity is underused [7]. The surgical mentor may not be a good teacher. In the OR, the teaching session cannot always be well designed or predicted. The case at hand may not be well suited for the learner. The progress or sequence of the operation cannot be altered to satisfy educational goals. Dissection and exposure cannot be performed for demonstration only. Steps may not be repeated, and the patient cannot be reassembled to start over if failure occurs [7]. In addition, fiscal constraints have resulted in pressure to achieve a high turnover in the OR, allowing less time for the attending staff to teach and trainees to practice skills [8]. Bridges and Diamond [8] have estimated that the annual cost of training chief residents in the OR amounts to more than $53 million per year, and suggest that adjunctive training environments that use traditional and virtual teachings aids may alleviate cost over time. In addition to time constraints, one cannot neglect the ethical issues of teaching and learning using patients [9].

There are tremendous advantages to training outside the OR. The learning environment is more easily controlled and adjusted. The learning situation can be tailored for each student's needs and can be altered on a minute-by-minute basis to create the desired effect. Perhaps the most valuable part of this training is granting "permission to fail" in a safe environment where there is no risk to patients. Studies have uncovered significant problems with the current surgical education curriculum. These include lack of continuity from undergraduate to graduate surgical education, and the lack of supervision when acquiring physical examination skill, ultimately resulting in poor performance [10–12]. An innovative educational tool, the Objective Structured Clinical Examination (OSCE) has proven useful in the evaluation of the clinical competence of surgical residents [13].

Surgical simulators have, perhaps, the best potential to mitigate surgical risk related to the educational process. A surgeon will be able to practice new procedures repeatedly until he or she is judged proficient without endangering patients. The surgeon can also be presented with cases of increasing complexity as his or her skills progress during training. Computer-based surgical simulators offer the potential for including operative cases representing all known anatomic variations. The training program director can use the simulator and its student tracking software to ensure that each graduating resident has seen and dealt with all the pertinent anatomic variations for that surgical specialty [14]. Using simulation, mistakes would lose their consequences and become ways to learn. A master surgeon's trick of the trade or critical maneuver during an operation could be learned in situ by every simulation user. The opportunity to learn something new this way has never before been available to medicine [15].

Another potential justification of virtual reality (VR) training is reducing the length of a surgical residency program. Currently, these training programs require five or more years in order to permit adequate exposure to a variety of technical procedures and decision-making situations. Training programs are currently time limited and not proficiency based. VR training could potentially reduce 5-year residency programs, because residents would not have to wait for clinical cases to appear. Instead, he or she could call up a variety of cases and perform the procedure in VR several times before doing so on a human [16]. One of the added attractions of simulation is that training programs might be able to correct for case-mix inequalities, so that what one learns in residency no longer depends only on what comes through the door when on call [15]. Flexibility is important for mastery of skills. Simulation may well offer the additional flexibility required. Though currently costly to implement on a large-scale, simulation offers great promise in future reduction of errors (and malpractice suites), reducing (or eliminating) the use of animals, and helping to establish standards for certain procedures.

An additional, and perhaps increasingly crucial, role of simulation may well be the assessment of possible decline in the skills of older surgeons. Measuring technical competence through VR could also be applied to older surgeons. As surgeons age, manual dexterity can decline, but it has always been difficult to objectively assess these skills. There is currently no mechanism to determine when these skill levels have deteriorated to the point where the surgeon should not be allowed to operate [16]. This decline in skills and judgment has traditionally been assessed by individual surgeons or chiefs of services. A mature, validated system of simulation-based education could offer for the first time a lifelong log of performance on standardized techniques, allowing measurement of skills independent of age or other arbitrary milestones [15].

6.2 Simulation and Simulators for Medical Education: Past, Present, and Future

VR is a computer-based, simulated environment in which users interact with a high-performance computer, graphics, specialized software, and devices providing visual, tactile, and auditory feedback, thereby simulating a true-life environment. VR-simulated environments allow trainees to repeat procedural experiences at their own leisure. These exercises or procedures would otherwise require numerous real-life encounters and costly hours of supervision [17].

A commonly recognized type of VR experience is that of flight simulation. In the aerospace, aviation, and defense industries, flight simulation is mandatory before pilots assume flight responsibilities. In addition, flight simulation is regularly used to help commercial airline pilots maintain their skills, or to become familiar with problems they might one day encounter.

Haluck et al. in 2001 [18] noted that virtual environments and computer-based simulators, although well-established training tools in other fields, have not been widely incorporated into surgical education. Concerns over the lack of validation, the cost, and finding time for residents to participate were cited as concerns. There are four major areas in medicine where VR is beginning to emerge: (1) assistance before and during medical surgical procedures, (2) medical education and training, (3) medical database visualization, and (4) rehabilitation [19].

For the most part, the advantages of flight simulators hold equally true for surgical simulators [19]. Surgical simulators can provide a concentrated environment that lends itself to learning complex tactile maneuvers in a relatively quick and proficient manner. Moreover, simulation of infrequent but highly hazardous events provides experience in handling these scenarios that may not be available during a period of routine flight or surgical training [20]. The ideal surgical simulator should provide the following: it can be customized to the needs of the student, the variety of cases during training increases significantly, and the student can chose to train only the difficult part of the surgery and repeat it as often as necessary [20].

Satava [19] has described five components that contribute to the realism of a virtual surgical world: fidelity, organ properties, organ reaction, interactivity, and sensory feedback. He predicts that the future holds promise of a virtual cadaver nearly indistinguishable from a real person [19]. This concept is referred to as the Turing test, a standard test that means to determine if a computer could be created that responds the way a human would respond such that a human could not tell the difference between the computer and a human [21, 22]. The VR Turing test would be met if an interrogating human could not tell the virtual human apart from the real human by sight, hearing, or touch, even dissection [20].

Current simulators do not yet meet the criteria of the Turing test. It is conceivable that future improvement in computing power and decreased costs of such technology will allow for development of such realism in a virtual environment. That being said, the level of fidelity required to meet the Turing test is likely not necessary to develop useful simulators that will teach useful skills in a validated fashion. In fact, many simulators are currently being used to teach medicine and range from low tech (inexpensive) to increasingly high tech, with corresponding price tags. The future use and development of simulation will depend in large part on validation of their effectiveness as training tools and to a certain extent the adoption of simulation by the various medical and surgical boards and societies. As organizations and institutions realize the potential cost savings (in dollars and lives) of training with simulation, investment from both private and public sources should follow.

Surgical skills laboratories have been successfully used for decades [10]. They were first introduced with simple tie-and-suture boards and pigskin suturing models in the 1960s [23]. Multiple tools and materials have been used since [24]. All of these skills laboratories require a clear curriculum and constructive feedback in order to be effective [25]. As one begins to organize a surgical skills center, the focus must be on curriculum with the choice of simulation and simulators based on fulfilling that curriculum.

Numerous simulators and VR training devices are currently available for training surgeons. Some of these are simple and inexpensive, while others are complex and costly. Simulators encompass everything from simple skills trainers such as knot-tying boards to part-task trainers such as a chest tube trainer, up to full procedural trainers that allow for training a complete laparoscopic or endoscopic procedure. Though by no means comprehensive, the following represents some of the types simulators that are currently available for teaching surgeons with a brief discussion of their utility (where applicable) for training.

6.2.1 Bench Models

Animal laboratory animal facilities are not accessible to all. Using animals to practice surgical procedures is prohibited in the United Kingdom. Martin et al. [26] have compared their open surgical bench models with performance of similar tasks in live anesthetized animals. Their correlations between scores on bench and live examinations were high, validating their bench models.

6.2.2 Laparoscopic Skills

The teaching of laparoscopic skills to surgeons has been a fertile ground for simulator development. One of the major reasons for this is that it is much easier to suspend the trainees' disbelief, as the actual procedure is done using long instruments while viewing a two-dimensional image on a monitor. Additionally, most of the haptics required is a result of movement of instruments through trocars, which is relatively easy to duplicate.

Fried et al. [27] have shown that performance by postgraduate year (PGY)-3 residents in an in vitro laparoscopic simulator correlated significantly with performance in an in vivo animal model. Likewise, practice in the simulator resulted in improved performance in vivo.

Hytlander et al. [28] have shown that training novice surgeons on the LapSim (Surgical Science) laparoscopic simulator translated to improved basic laparoscopic skill performance in a porcine model, suggesting that skills learned on a simulator can be transferred to the OR.

Scott et al. [29] demonstrated that junior surgical residents who had formal laparoscopic skills training had improved operative performance with laparoscopic cholecystectomy more than did their nontrained peers.

In an important article in 2002, Seymour et al. [30] validated the transfer of training skills from VR to OR, by showing that residents who were pretrained to "expert criterion" on the Minimally Invasive Surgical Trainer – Virtual Reality (MIST-VR) performed better in the OR than did their non–VR-trained counterparts, with significantly less failure to progress, injury to gallbladder, burning of non–target tissue, and fewer errors. This was one of the first studies to demonstrate that individuals who train on a simulator can translate those skills into improved performance and outcome, a finding that should help further ignite enthusiasm (and funding) for skills training centers.

6.2.3 Gastrointestinal Endoscopy

Endoscopic procedures have also been fertile ground for development of high-fidelity simulators. As with laparoscopy, these procedures entail interaction with a patient through an instrument (the scope) with visualization on a monitor. For more than 30 years, different types of simulators, including mechanical [31], animal [32], animal-part [33], and computer-based models [34] have been used to teach and learn endoscopic procedures. The goals of simulator-based teaching methods should be the acceleration and improvement of training in endoscopy for beginners, the maintenance of competency with endoscopic procedures, and testing of new procedures prior to performance on a patient [35].

One such virtual endoscopy simulator (GI-Mentor, Simbionix, Tel Hashomer, Israel) has been shown to be capable of identifying differences between beginners and experts in gastrointestinal endoscopy. Training on this simulator for 3 weeks improved performance of beginners significantly in a study conducted by Fer-

litsch et al. in 2002 [35]. In a separate study, Ritter et al. [36] have shown that the GI Mentor simulator can distinguish between novice and intermediate endoscopists. They concluded that the simulator assesses skills with levels of consistency and reliability required for high-stakes assessment.

6.2.4 Endonasal Surgery

Edmond [37] reported that training residents on an endoscopic sinus surgical simulator had a positive impact on OR performance among junior otolaryngology residents. In contrast, Caversaccio and colleagues [38] reported that an endonasal surgery simulator allowed junior surgical trainees to better understand the anatomy, but failed to make an impact on OR performance. They cited some of the limitations of the particular simulator, including absence of force feedback and considerable time consumption.

6.2.5 Urology

Matsumoto [39] demonstrated a positive effect of training at the surgical skills laboratory on endourological skills. Jacomedies et al. have suggested that virtual ureterscopy simulator training may allow beginning urology residents to shorten the initial learning curve associated with ureteroscopy training [40].

6.2.6 Bronchoscopy

Bronchoscopy training on a simulator readily includes deliberate action, reaction, opportunities for repetition, correction of errors, and ability for individualized learning, all key components to the educational process [5]. Rowe and Cohen [41] demonstrated that training on a bronchoscopy simulator translated into improved performance on subsequent fiber optic intubation in children.

6.2.7 Anesthesiology

No other specialty to date has embraced simulation as actively as has anesthesiology. The emphasis has been on team training and crisis management more than on specific skills.

Chopra et al. [42] demonstrated that anesthesiologists trained on a high-fidelity anesthesia simulator responded more quickly and appropriately when handling a crisis on a simulator. Controlled studies involving humans to validate this finding would present an unacceptable risk, however. Further development of the simulation concept evolved out of the recognition that two thirds of all accidents or incidents in anesthesia can be attributed to human error. To counter this, Howard and colleagues [43] developed a training program entitled Anesthesia Crisis Resource Management in order to optimize anesthesiologist and team performance during stressful incidents. Success in this arena has led to the use of mannequin-based simulators in surgical training as an alternative to "real" trauma resuscitations for teaching teamwork and crisis-management skills [10, 44].

Several other simulators are currently available or under development for a variety of medical specialties. It is beyond the scope of this chapter to present these in detail. Suffice it to say that more of these will become available with increasing realism and sophistication in the very near future. Perhaps the greatest lesson to be learned as we utilize these new technologies is that although VR enhances training, it does not replace existing methodology. A considered synthesis of the two, however, inevitably requires that we redefine the idea of what constitutes a complete medical education.

VR systems introduce the alluring possibility of a completely objective measurement and assessment of the trainee's ability. As the cost of simulators is still quite high, very few institutions can afford to obtain and maintain a large inventory that may be necessary to meet the needs of all surgical learners. As such, the idea of regional centers makes sense. The exact makeup of such a center will depend in large part on the needs of the learners and the resources available. The most logical approach to developing such a skills center is to identify the population to be trained, the skills that they need, and then develop robust curriculum to meet those needs. Only then should consideration be given to what simulators to purchase to meet those needs.

In other words, the curriculum should dictate the simulators and not vice versa. The remainder of this chapter is devoted to looking at a case study of how one institution has responded to the challenge of training for disruptive technologies by constructing a comprehensive simulation center. This example is by no means meant to be prescriptive, but will hopefully serve as an example of things that must be considered when organizing such a center.

6.2.8   Case Study: The National Capital Area Medical Simulation Center

The National Capital Area Medical Simulation Center (NCAMSC) is part of the Uniformed Services University of the Health Sciences (the United States' only military medical school) located in Bethesda, Maryland. Officially opened in April of 2000, the Center uses a variety of medical simulation approaches and technologies to teach and evaluate clinical and surgical skills. Its target population consists of medical and nursing students, interns and residents, and practicing physicians. The NCAMSC is the first single location to integrate the use of VR technology, computer-controlled mannequins, and human-simulated patients under one roof. The Center is contained in roughly 11,000 contiguous square feet and is divided into four functional areas. The floor plan of the center is shown in Figure 6.1.

The Center is divided into four functional areas. These are the Administrative Area, the Clinical Assessment Laboratory, the Computer Laboratory, and the Surgical Simulation Laboratory. Each distinct area can sustain educational activities on its own, and when necessary integrate the operations of the entire Center for a more comprehensive approach. All of the functional areas have been designed to maximize students' access to clinical experience in a state-of-the-art learning environment.

6.2.8.1   The Administrative Area

The administrative area of NCAMSC is the hub of the Center. It incorporates the administrative offices as well as the video teleconference room or VTC Room.

The Administrative Area serves as the hub for daily operational concerns such as personnel, budgeting, and resource allocation. This area houses the offices of the Center to include the medical director, the director of clinical skills/standardized patient training, and the administrative director.

The VTC is the Center's audio/video entry and exit point to the outside world (Fig. 6.2) Equipped with state-of-the art video teleconferencing equipment, any of the video signals from around the center can be routed through this room and sent to all connected sites anywhere in the world. This allows remote sites to participate and review many of the exercises that take place in the center.

This room is also equipped with a "telecommuting" conference table, which allows up to 12 students, faculty, or visitors to connect their laptops to any of the 12 local area network ports for high-speed Internet access. The table is also outfitted with 16 headphone ports, allowing various audio exercises that permit instructors and students to sample the same audio files simultaneously for review and discussion. As a standard conference room, it is also equipped with slide-to-video converter, document camera, and VCR.

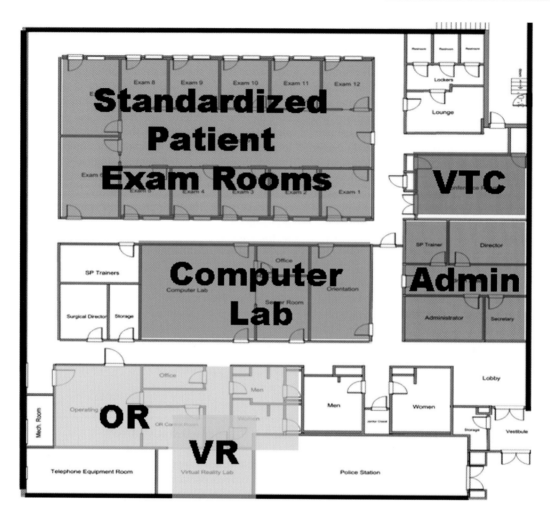

Fig. 6.1 The floor plan of the National Capital Area Medical Simulation Center. The Center contains a video teleconferencing suite (VTC), an administrative area, a virtual reality (VR) lab, a virtual operating room (OR), a 16-station computer lab, and a 12-room standardized patient exam area with a central control/monitoring area

6.2.8.2 Clinical Assessment Laboratory

The clinical assessment laboratory is designed for teaching and evaluating students in the basic clinical skills of history taking, physical examination, communication, and interpersonal skills. Here simulated patient encounters provide an ideal transition from the classroom to real patient contact. The clinical assessment laboratory also prepares students for the US Medical Licensure Examination. An additional three standardized patient trainers are employed to ensure the smooth operation of this area. This area consists of four sub sections.

The Orientation Room is used to brief students. Ceiling-mounted, drop-screen and LCD projectors are used to display PowerPoint and/or video presentations for orientation, registration, and briefing the students on specific event protocols. Here students are registered for clinical events through a login process that tracks them throughout their activities.

The Clinical Exam Room Area consists of 12 exam rooms that serve as the simulated clinical environment. There are ten regular (120 NSF) exam rooms and two large (220 NSF) rooms with hospital beds that can be used for inpatient and/or critical care simulation. The large rooms are also suited for trauma simulation and small-group teaching events.

In the Clinical Exam Room Area, students have the opportunity for live patient encounters that simulate specific challenges in outpatient, inpatient, or critical care settings (Fig. 6.3). Specifically, individuals (referred to as standardized patients) are hired and trained

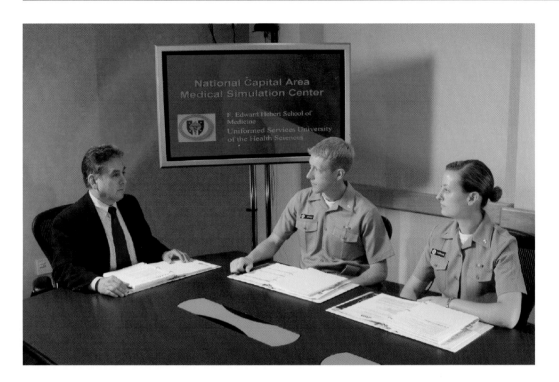

Fig. 6.2 The Video Teleconferencing Room (VTC) of the National Capital Area Medical Simulation Center

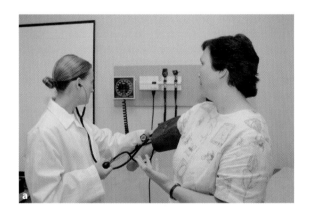
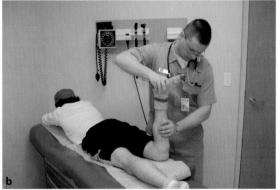

Fig. 6.3 Clinical Exam Rooms in the National Capital Area Medical Simulation Center. Here "standardized" patients are being examined by medical students

to simulate scripted clinical cases. These clinical cases may be simulated using performance, make-up, or real conditions and sometimes a combination of all three.

Each exam room is equipped with two video cameras and microphones that permit encounters to be recorded for subsequent analysis. Each room also contains a computer for each patient and a wall-mounted computer located outside of the room for each student to use for pre- and post-encounter documentation.

Typically, clinical exams are designed following a directive to achieve specific educational goals. The standardized patient trainers and the medical director collaborate with faculty members to create projects that meet stated educational goals.

The Monitoring Area is at the center of the Clinical Exam Room Area and allows the standardized patient trainer and faculty instructors to monitor the progress of clinical exams. A specialized video router controls

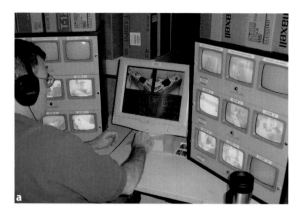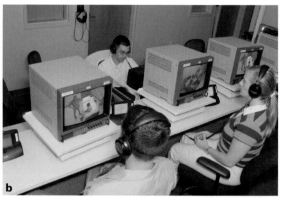

Fig. 6.4 **a** The control panel that allows for optimal positioning of the camera's in the patient exam room. **b** The central monitoring area allows faculty to view single or multiple rooms from one location

24 videotape decks that track students as they move from room to room. A touch-screen control panel permits cameras to be positioned for optimal imaging (Fig. 6.4). Faculty and students are able to view the encounter through one-way mirrors outside each room or from central monitors that allow monitoring of multiple rooms simultaneously (Fig. 6.4). Faculty and students may also review and learn from recorded tapes as if they were in the room, allowing for more detailed observation and dynamic feedback. The monitoring area is also used for training simulated patients.

The Standardized Patient Lounge is a staging area for simulated and standardized patients to prepare and relax. This area is required as patients often use theatrical makeup to simulate traumatic injuries or other conditions.

6.2.8.3 Computer Laboratory

The Computer Laboratory has two sections, the Computer Laboratory itself and an adjacent Control Room.

The Computer Laboratory has two primary functions. The first is to identify, develop, and/or use medical education software that contributes toward clinical or medical readiness skills. The second is to provide an environment in which computer-based, interactive clinical examinations can be administered (Fig. 6.5).

The Computer Laboratory consists of 16 Internet-accessible workstations that run a variety of medical educational CD ROMs. Eight overhead cameras and a one-way mirror between the Lab and the Computer Control room ensure that examinations can be properly monitored when the Lab is used for testing. Students use the computer laboratory to work with interactive

software programs that may be linked to activities occurring in other functional areas of the Center.

Additionally, students can prepare for the NMBE (National Board of Medical Examiners) exam by practicing test questions from several test prep software packages available in the center. Currently, the computer lab meets or exceeds the requirements to be a NBME testing site. Students and faculty can also use the computers to conduct independent studies or view university mail or class schedules.

The Computer Control Room is adjacent to the Computer Laboratory. It is the nerve center of the Center. All data, voice, and video signals are fed through the Control Room and can be routed to other areas accordingly. The Control Room also houses several departmental servers that handle the current needs of the center.

During testing, the Control Room operates as a monitoring station for instructors, allowing overall viewing of the Computer Laboratory through the one-way mirrored window or any of the workstations individually from the overhead camera. A high-speed fiber optic link between the Center and the National Library of Medicine also exists. This link provides the Center with access to Internet II, which is still in the development stage. This link will be used to test and develop streaming video and other high-bandwidth/high-reliability applications as they are developed to augment medical training.

6.2.8.4 Surgical Simulation Laboratory

The Surgical Simulation Laboratory uses VR and a full-scale OR mock-up to provide highly realistic scenarios for surgical training. This area was the

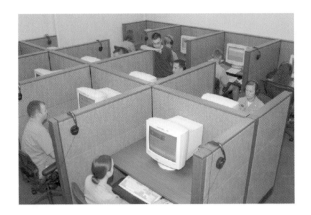

Fig. 6.5 The Computer Lab of the National Capital Area Simulation Center. The Lab consists of 16 PC workstations

first site approved to investigate teaching the surgical skills practicum of the Advanced Trauma Life Support course, using computer-based simulators and plastic models rather than anesthetized animals or cadavers.

The Operating Room (O.R.) is furnished to look and feel like a typical OR. In addition to the typical O.R. equipment, the room holds intravenous catheterization, endoscopy, and diagnostic ultrasound simulators. The O.R. can be configured to match the conditions of a standard O.R., an emergency room or an intensive care unit. Here, three human-patient simulators that respond to various drugs and interventions are used for teaching medical and surgical interventions and teamwork to a variety of health care providers (Fig. 6.6).

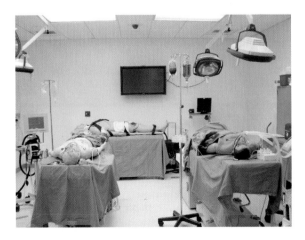

Fig. 6.6 The Operating Room of the National Capital Area Medical Simulation Center, showing three high-fidelity human-patient simulators (*foreground*) and an ultrasound simulator in the *back right corner*

Driven by computers, the human-patient simulators can be preprogrammed with patient characteristics or variables such as age, anatomy, and physiology factors, depending on the training event. Students are faced with real-life situations as they interact with the human simulator, depending on the scripted clinical procedure. The simulators have palpable pulse areas and will exhibit the appropriate physiologic reactions in response to various intravenous or inhaled agents. The simulators can be moulaged to represent wounds and clinical conditions (Fig. 6.7). Presently, one of the simulators has the capability for 80 different drugs to be "virtually" administered by various computer microchips. The simulator responds to the type and amount of these drugs according to instructor-determined, preprogrammed patient variables. The simulators provide a very powerful tool teaching a variety of clinical scenarios. The O.R. is staffed by a full time coordinator and a physician surgical director, whose offices are also found in this area.

In the O.R. Control Room, overhead microphones, four overhead video cameras, and a one-way mirror into the O.R. allow instructors to communicate with the O.R. coordinator. In the Control Room, the coordinator can change patient variables on the computer and even speak into a hidden microphone feed on the simulated patients in order to bring more realism to the scene. An additional feature in the control room is a button that will turn off the power in the O.R., allowing for the simulation of what to do during a real power outage (Fig. 6.8).

The Virtual Reality (VR) Laboratory develops and tests computer-based surgical simulators to meet the educational objectives of the Center. Research that advances simulation procedures is also a fundamental directive as is harnessing the capabilities of existing technologies. This area is also run by the surgical director with a staff that includes a Ph.D. computer scientist, software developers, and a graphic artist. In the VR Laboratory, state-of-the-art computer-based equipment enables students to view medical objects in two or three dimensions. A haptic interface allows the computers to recreate the tactile sense that permits users to touch, feel, manipulate, create, and alter simulated three-dimensional anatomic structures in a virtual environment. Here students can teach themselves at their own pace and can feel comfortable about making mistakes as well as repeating an exercise. The VR Laboratory is equipped with simulators for vascular anastomosis, laparoscopic surgery, bronchoscopy, pericardiocentesis, a diagnostic peritoneal lavage unit, and a hand-immersive environment for on-going research (Fig. 6.9). Both the pericardiocentesis and diagnostic peritoneal lavage simulators were developed in the VR Laboratory. These two simulators are the first of their kind and are unique to the Center. The VR Laboratory

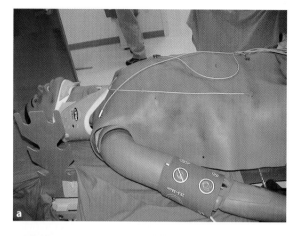

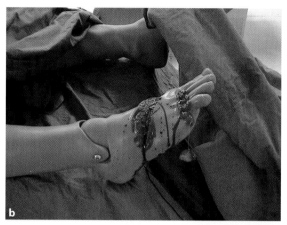

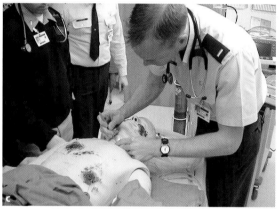

Fig. 6.7 Moulaged high-fidelity human-patient simulators. **a** A blunt trauma scenario with a "seatbelt sign," **b** a mangled extremity, **c** a patient with gunshot wounds across face and the chest receiving a surgical airway, **d** the same patient being electrocardioverted for an arrhythmia

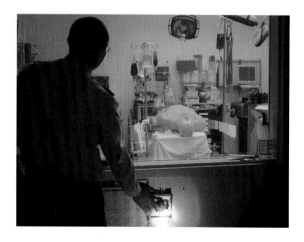

Fig. 6.8 A view of the Operating Room from the Control Room through the one-way mirror. The red button on the wall turns off the power in the Operating Room to allow for team training under such circumstances

is actively involved in ongoing validation research of existing and newly developed simulators, and continues to take the lead in developing new simulators and simulation technology.

6.3   Conclusion

For reasons of educational quality, safety, and cost, VR and simulation can enhance surgical training and learning now, and their role will almost certainly expand as computer power and availability increase. Clearly, the introduction of simulation into medical education is a disruptive force that challenges the status quo. However, it is likely that societal pressure to reduce errors in the face of decreased time and availability of clinical teaching material will result in mandates to provide training and maintenance of skills using simulation. Forward-thinking institutions should embrace the

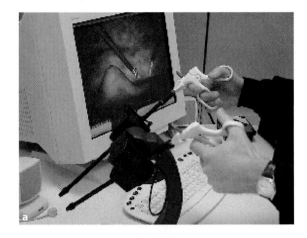

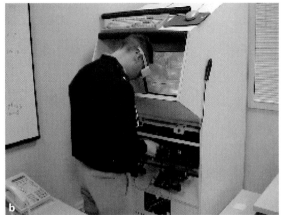

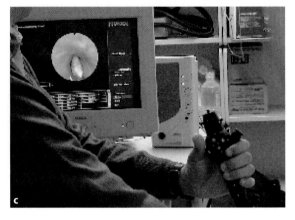

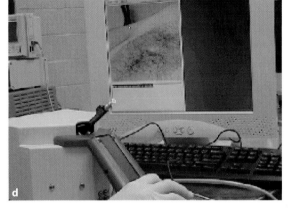

Fig. 6.9 Examples of virtual reality simulators found in the VR lab at the National Capital Area Medical Simulation Center. **a** Laparoscopic surgery simulator, **b** vascular anastomosis simulator, **c** bronchoscopy simulator, and **d** diagnostic peritoneal lavage simulator

adoption of simulation in well–thought out curriculum that will meet the educational needs of the learners that they support. Careful thought should be given to how resources should be spent and centers organized to respond to the present and future challenges. It is essential that centers should be built with flexibility in mind and should be staffed with a full complement of educators, clinicians, and administrative and support personnel. Ideally, centers will also engage in validation research and development of simulators and curricula that will continue to push this exciting and rapidly growing field ever forward to respond to future disruptive technologies as they occur.

References

1. Russell T (2003) From my perspective. Bull Am Coll Surg 88:3–4

2. Sternberg S (2004) Science clearing the way for shift in fighting stroke. USA Today. http://www.usatoday. com/tech/news/techinovations/2004-04-26-stents-strokes.

3. Kohn LT, Corrigan JM, Donaldson MS (eds.) (2000) To err is human: building a safer health system. Committee on Quality of Health Care in America, Institute of Medicine. National Academy Press, Washington, D.C.

4. Kaufman DM, Bell W (1997) Teaching and assessing clinical skills using virtual reality. Medicine meets virtual reality. Morgan KS et al (eds.) IOS, Amsterdam, pp 467–472

5. Colt HG, Crawford SW, Galbraith O (2001) Virtual reality bronchoscopy simulation: a revolution in procedural training. Chest 120:1333–1339

6. Haluck RS, Krummel TM (2000) Computers and virtual reality for surgical education in the 21st century. Arch Surg 135:786–792

7. Scallon SE, Fairholm DJ, Cochrane DD, Taylor DC (2001) Evaluation of the operating room as a teaching venue. Can J Surg 35:173–176

8. Bridges M, Diamond DL (1999) The financial impact of teaching surgical residents in the operating room. Am J Surg 177:28–32

9. Gates EA (1997) New surgical procedures: can our patients benefit while we learn? Am J Obstet Gynecol 176:1293–1297

10. Gorman PJ, Meier AH, Krummel TM (2000) Computer-assisted training and learning in surgery. Comp Aid Surg 5:120–130

11. Chalabian J, Garman K, Wallace P, Dunnington G (1996) Clinical breast evaluation skills of house officers and students. Am Surg 62:840–845

12. Endean ED, Sloan DA, Veldenz HC, Donnelly MB, Schwarcz TH (1994) Performance of the vascular physical examination by residents and medical students. J Vasc Surg 19:149–156

13. Sloan DA, Donnelly MB, Schwartz RW, Strodel WE (1995) The objective structured clinical examination. The new gold standard for evaluating postgraduate clinical performance. Ann Surg 222:735–742

14. Kaufmann CR (2001) Computers in surgical education and the operating room. Ann Chir Gynaecol 90:141–143

15. Dawson SL (2002) A critical approach to medical simulation. Bull Am Coll Surg 87:12–18

16. Ota D, Loftin B, Saito T, Lea R, Keller J (1995) Virtual reality in surgical education. Comput Biol Med 25:127–137

17. Issenberg SB, McGeghie WC, Hart IR et al (1999) Simulation technology for health care professional skills training and assessment. JAMA 282:861–867

18. Haluck RS, Marshall RL, Krummel TM, Melkonian MG (2001) Are surgery training programs ready for virtual reality? A survey of program directors in general surgery. J Am Coll Surg 193:660–665

19. Satava RM (1995) Medical applications of virtual reality. J Med Syst 19:275–280

20. Lange T, Indelicato DJ, Rosen JM (2000) Virtual reality in surgical training. Surg Oncol Clin N Am 9:61–79

21. Bleich HL, Turing A (1995) The machine, the enigma, and the test. MD Comput 12:330–334

22. Heiser JF, Colby KM, Faught WS et al (1979) Can psychiatrists distinguish a computer simulation of paranoia from the real thing? The limitations of Turing-like test measures of the adequacy of simulation. J Psychiatr Res 15:149–162

23. Boyle DE, Gius JA (1968) Tie and suture training board. Surgery 63:434–436

24. Gorman PJ, Meier AH, Krummel TM (1999) Simulation and virtual reality in surgical education: real or unreal? Arch Surg 134:1203–1208

25. Barnes RW, Lange NP, Whiteside MF (1989) Halstedian technique revisited. Innovations in teaching surgical skills. Ann Surg 210:1187–1121

26. Martin JA, Regehr G, Reznick R, Macrae H, Murnahan J, Hutchinson C, Brown M (1997) Objective structured assessment of technical skill (OSATS) for surgical residents. Br J Surg 84:273–278

27. Fried GM, Derossis AM, Bothwell J, Sigman HH (1999) Comparison of laparoscopic performance in vivo with performance measured in a laparoscopic simulator. Surg Endosc 13:1077–1081

28. Hyltander A, Liljegren E, Rhondin PH, Lönroth H (2002) The transfer of basic skills learned in a laparoscopic simulator to the operating room. Surg Endosc 16:1324–1328

29. Scott DJ, Bergen PC, Rege RV, Laycock R, Tesfay ST, Valentine RJ, Euhus DM, Jeyarajah DR, Thompson WM, Jones DB (2000) Laparoscopic training on bench models: better and more cost effective than operating room experience. J Am Coll Surg 191:272–283

30. Seymour NE, Gallagher AG, Roman SA, O'Brien MK, Bansal VK, Anderson DK, Satava RM (2002) Virtual reality training improves operating room performance: results of a randomized, double-blinded study. Ann Surg 236:458–464

31. Markman HD (1969) A new system for teaching proctosigmoidoscopic morphology. Am J Gastroenterol 52:65–69

32. Noar MD (1995) An established porcine model for animate training in diagnostic and therapeutic ERCP. Endoscopy 27:77–80

33. Freys SM, Heimbucher J, Fuchs KH (1995) Teaching upper gastrointestinal endoscopy: the pig stomach. Endoscopy 27:73–76

34. Bar-Meir S (2000) A new endoscopic simulator. Endoscopy 32:898–900

35. Ferlitsch A, Glauninger P, Gupper A, Schillinger M, Haefner M, Gangl A, Schoefl R (2002) Evaluation of a virtual endoscopy simulator for training in gastrointestinal endoscopy. Endoscopy 34:698–702

36. Ritter EM, McClusky DA, Lederman AB, Gallagher AG, Smith CD (2003) Objective psychomotor skills assessment of experienced and novice flexible endoscopists with a virtual reality simulator. J Gastrointest Surg 7:871–878

37. Edmond CV (2002) Impact of the endoscopic sinus surgical simulator on operating room performance. Laryngoscope 112:1148–1158

38. Caversaccio M, Eichenberger A, Häusler R (2003) Virtual simulator as a training tool for endonasal surgery. Am J Rhinology 17:283–290

39. Matsumoto ED, Hamstra SJ, Radomski SB, Cusimano MD (2001) A novel approach to endosurgical training: training at the Surgical Skills Center. J Urology 166:1261–1266

40. Jacomides L, Ogan K, Cadeddu JA, Pearle MS (2004) Use of a virtual reality simulator for ureteroscopy training. J Urology 171:320–323

41. Rowe R, Cohen RA (2002) An evaluation of a virtual reality airway simulator. Anesth Analg 95:62–66

42. Chopra V, Gesink BJ, de Jong J, Bovill JG, Spierdijk J, Brand R (1994) Does training on an anesthesia simulator lead to improvement in performance? Br J Anaest 73:293–297

43. Howard S, Gaba D, Fish K, Yang G, Sarnquist F (1992) Anesthesia crisis resource management training: teaching anesthesiologists to handle critical incidents. Aviat Space Environ Med 63:763–770

44. McLellan BA (1999) Early experience with simulated trauma resuscitation. Can J Surg 42:205–210

Ideal VR systems: Is There a „Holy Grail" in Simulation System Land?

7

Nicola Di Lorenzo

Since the Middle Ages and until today, the education of surgeons has always consisted of "learning on the job." In the daily practice of surgical residency all over the world, a large part of surgical skills is still learned in the operating room while working on patients. However, learning on human beings is not always the best way, not for the patient nor for the surgical trainee. All residency programs are reducing working hours for trainees; the introduction of new technologies and the minimally invasive revolution have certainly increased the number and sometimes the complexity of procedures; ethical considerations have led us to nearly abandon the use of cadavers for enhancing surgical experience, while animal labs are strongly contrasted in most Western countries. These issues elicit the need to develop alternative training methods using physical models, box trainers, or electronic simulators.

While thinking that we are living in a very advanced and technological era, we must keep in mind that iatrogenic pathology is nowadays the seventh cause of death. Therefore, recognition of the importance of errors is an essential component of the practice of surgery, and new methods and technologies are being used to identify, avoid, and reduce errors. The medical community in general has ascribed errors to the system; however, during a surgical procedure, surgeons are the only actors of an error, and the consequences are more and more relevant, considering that litigation is a main issue as well.

The possibility of reducing medical errors (surgical acts account for 50% of them) could then dramatically influence the healthcare systems, and socioeconomic advantages could be at least as relevant as they were 30 years ago, when flight simulators introduced as a standardized part of the curriculum of in-training pilot brought a 30% reduction in civil aviation accidents.

Many new methods to train surgeons have become available as education, training, and accurate assessment of skill and performance represent the most important challenge of the new century for medical schools, scientific societies, academic and clinical environments.

Two main examples are mentioned:

1. In his presidential address at the Society of American Gastrointestinal and Endoscopic Surgeons (SAGES) 2002 Meeting, William L. Traverso said that the three missions of SAGES for the 3rd millennium are "Education, education, and … education!" Before and after this statement, SAGES has dedicated major resources and efforts to this goal.
2. At the same time, the European Association for Endoscopic Surgery (EAES) created in 2004 the Work Group for Evaluation and Implementation of Simulators and Skills Training programs, thus devoting intellectual and financial resources to these new educational opportunities.

Medical education, a field where tradition has always played a main role, is now introducing a "bits-and-bytes" system with the use of information technology, thus undergoing significant changes. Simulators have achieved widespread acceptance in the field of anesthesia, intensive care, flexible endoscopy, and recently in surgery, especially for minimally invasive surgery. The fast introduction of minimally invasive skills has speeded up the development of new training methods to train residents through these new technologies.

Some simulators are based on phantoms (physical models, e.g., plastic structures) others are virtual reality (VR) computer-based simulators. A third group is represented by the hybrid simulators, where the two components are integrated (Fig. 7.1).

Although phantoms may provide realism concerning tissue behavior, computer-based simulators will increasingly become more eligible as a training aid, especially because of their extensive range of educational features. Several systems are on the market, and producers are continuously enhancing their products, covering the field of more popular procedures with virtual reconstructions. In some recent studies, although evidence-based validation is not yet achieved, it has been shown that they can improve surgeons' performance, predicting a significant contribution to patient care.

physical	VR	HYBRID
• Simulab • MATT • 3-D technical service • Medina trainer • LCSAD	• Xitact • Simbionix • METI SEP • VEST; select-it • Accutouch-Immersion • Lapsim • Mentice • SIMENDO-DeltaTech	• Promis-Haptica • Realsim • CELTS-Medicalsim

Fig. 7.1 Simulators on the market

Key points and advantages of VR simulation can be summarized as follows:
- Long periods of training without the physical presence of a tutor
- Large number of simulations and exercises
- Repetition of the scenery
- Flexibility of the scenery
- Score system for evaluation and learning assessment
- Network of models: net connections to exchange information for the development of teaching and learning
- New pedagogy and better motivation, representing the meeting point between professional education and the "PlayStation generation," using the positive impact of the so-called videogame effect

When considering simulator design, a complete understanding of several aspects, including human learning, human factors, technology, and the field of simulation in general, is required. Development requires expertise in surgery, education, computer graphics (and possibly haptics), computer programming in general, and in simulation technology. In the pioneering days of surgical simulation in early 1990s, most developers did not apply a comprehensive approach, and it is now clear that simulators created without a thorough knowledge of these areas are unlikely to be useful in today's teaching process.

Moreover, the knowledge of the learning process must be very well interpreted, as learning theories play a determinant role in the transfer of learning on models to the real procedures.

We want to stress here two main points:
1. The most commonly used theories to explain human learning are based on constructivism. A continuous increase in knowledge or change in behavior is brought about through "learning by doing" or "experiential learning" (Kolb). If we speed up this

process, a faster and more reliable education can be achieved.
2. It is equally important to remember that surgical simulation is a very reliable application for the model of Rasmussen, who distinguished three levels of human behavior:
   a. Skill-based behavior (SBB)
   b. Rule-based behavior (RBB)
   c. Knowledge-based behavior (KBB)

It indicates that different training simulators need to be developed related to different behavior levels (Fig. 7.2). At the lower level (SBB), simulators are needed to learn basic skills, such as using instruments. For higher-level training (RBB and KBB), surgical skill improvement requires more sophisticated training methods. For example, to enhance patient safety by reducing human errors and critical and unexpected situations (e.g., power failure, instrument breakdown), trainees should be trained at the knowledge-based behavior level.

The potential of learning via multimedia resources must be finally stressed. The commonest form of audiovisual link is a broadband connection that can be easily used between the operating room and the surgical skills center and, with the development of the "intelligent OR," audio-\visual information to and from the operating room can be integrated with the system. Simulation can then be performed on real cases, responding positively to the criticism on the transfer from VR to real practice. Equally important is the chance, thanks to powerful audiovisual requirements, to broadcast simulation sessions from one skills centre to the other, increasing a network of models running on the same digital platform.

Validity and reliability of simulators are key points for their validation as educational tools. This explains why educators and simulation experts must learn and imbed new words in their cultural knowledge, such as

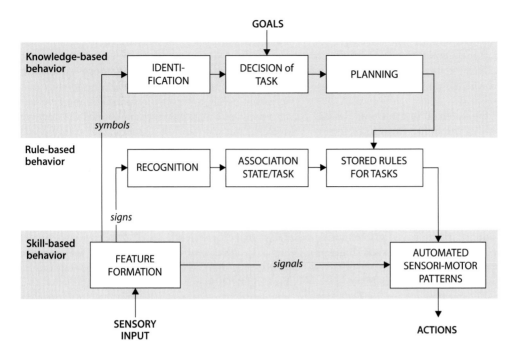

Fig. 7.2 The Rasmussen model

taxonomy and metrics. The Virtual Reality Turing Test, Objective Structured Clinical Exam (OSCE), Objective Structured Assessment of Technical Skills (OSATS), McGill Inanimate System for Training and Evaluation of Laparoscopic Skills (MISTELS), and Minimally Invasive Surgical Training – Virtual Reality (MIST-VR) are examples of evaluation modalities based on these parameters.

In this regard, it is of utmost importance the work of the aforementioned Work Group for Evaluation and Implementation of Simulators and Skills Training programs of EAES, based on following a systematic process to establish minimal requirements and get to a standardized model for simulator's validation, using literature meta-analysis, testing, and guidelines creation.

Summarizing the above-depicted characteristics and potentials of simulators, one could imagine that no major obstacle blocks the road of wide diffusion as the main revolution in surgical education of the modern era. This is not true, as these tools belong to a newborn market, and producers are facing major problems in terms of fidelity and realism, reproducibility of true procedures, technological limitations, and clear validation of their effectiveness in transfer the acquired skills to clinical practice.

The use of effective virtual models means to interact with them, in a VR environment, exerting on them traction and forces. This interaction requires perceptive interfaces (visual, acoustical, tactile), in order to

make immersive virtual environments suitable for human senses.

The main limits of simulators for general surgery in the current state-of-the-art can be summarized as follows:

- Realistic interaction with a virtual model
- Touch
- Force
- Complex anatomy
- Organs variability
- Several conditions of pathology and development of that for surgical therapy
- Movement variability
- Thickness of organs and tissues
- External forces

From this list, two main critical points are addressed:

1. There is still a lot of effort needed to implement these VR systems with a better realistic haptics and tactile feedback: They are currently mediated by complex devices, or they reproduced by smart but simpler technologies that mimic them through frictions or other physical methods. The results are not yet very satisfactory, as they are not for robots used for telesurgery in clinical practice.
2. Lack of realism in simulation of tissue properties is another important limit, as changes induced by pathological conditions (inflammation, scarring, sclerosis, vascularization, etc.) bring to an enormous

variability. Several complex mathematical models have been introduced, not yet with a satisfactory result. Probably, the solution will come with the enhanced computational ability of computers that is exponentially growing up since their introduction.

The recognition of the potential of electronic devices brings the argument of the utility of introducing robotic technology in the simulation devices. Currently, as Satava has stated, surgical robots are nothing other than computers with arms, as a Tc-scan is a computer with eyes, etc. Integrating them into an intelligent OR is a main goal of clinical application of technology. The same integration will bring to 3D VR for learning and practice, with the opportunity to have flexible models, representing the anatomic variations of each single patient and looking at anatomic organs from perspectives that would be impossible during surgery. This will dramatically enhance the educational capacities of simulation, amplifying the surgeon's dexterity through the use of suitable haptic and robotic interfaces. In facts, they will become more and more useful in repeating and electronically comparing training programs, remote teaching, and preoperative planning on virtual patients, and in performing specific diagnostic and therapeutic procedures.

7.1   Curriculum

Learning through VR simulation modalities is not yet being systematically introduced in the curricula of the residency programs in European countries (actually,

the Royal College of Surgeons has a defined program, and the Royal College of Surgeons of Ireland is planning a selection of candidates for residency programs including attitudinal evaluation through simulation, but nothing has been standardized, i.e., in Italy and Germany), while a rational approach in the field has started in Unite States (American Council of Graduate Medical Education and the American Board of Medical Specialties).

The creation of reliable predictive tests, based on VR simulation, to assess candidate's attitude to surgery will represent an additional criterion to be integrated with other attitudinal evaluations for the access to the residency programs. Although still under debate, the prediction of proficiency based on Cuschieri's model (Fig. 7.3) could save relevant resources and increase health care safety, contemporarily addressing unsuitable candidates to nonsurgical specialties.

Scientific society must play the main role in managing, standardizing, and correctly addressing this evolution, quickly understanding that the change in surgical teaching needs to be driven by independent and noncommercial authorities. It is then necessary in the near future to establish an international consensus for an integrated curriculum, not only for surgeon training, but also to assess periodically the skill maintenance of surgeons in clinical activity. It must be remembered that, without the introduction of minimally invasive procedures, most surgeons have not had the chance to receive complete training before applying the laparoscopic technique to their patients, and this is very evident by the increased percentage of lesions (e.g., of the biliary tree) present in the learning curve of a generation. This will not be acceptable in the future,

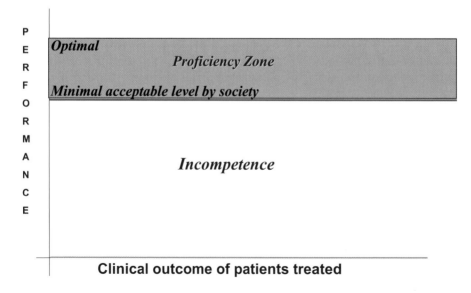

Fig. 7.3 Cuschieri's model of proficiency

when reliable simulation will elevate a surgeon's skill, increasing the patients' safety.

Simulation and attitudinal evaluation, at a lower level, could be used as well for medical schools students' selection, using the same productivity criteria applied to simpler tasks for novices.

Finally, another field of application for the satisfactory VR simulator of the future is the possibility of testing and evaluating new instruments: New tools and innovative technologies can be tested while still in a computer-animated design (CAD) configuration, increasing safety and significantly reducing costs. Following the same guidelines, new surgical techniques will be safely introduced and mastered on virtual patients before being introduced in clinical practice.

Now, the question introduced in the title can be slightly but significantly modified: Is there a "holy grail" in the described simulation systems? Is it possible, at the state-of-the-art point where we are now, to say when a multifunctional system will be able to cover satisfactorily all needs of a comprehensive program for trainees?

Current experience is negative, but future developments, although challenging, can bridge the gap, giving us the chance to change today's negative answer in a future's positive one.

Apart from the already-described and well-known pitfalls of simulation systems, there are more general consideration to be introduced:

- Development of simulators is currently devoted almost completely to laparoscopic surgery and minimally invasive techniques, such as endovascular procedures. It is evident that medical treatments will be increasingly performed with a less invasive approach; nevertheless, it is equally clear that, at least in the future of current generations, a large amount of procedures will be still completed with a traditional techniques, especially in the fields of emergency or major procedures. Moreover, some of these complex operations will not be planned, but will represent the rescue treatment of complications occurred during minimally invasive surgery. As a third important aspect, the surgeon generation trained after the 1980 is brilliantly skilled in laparoscopic complex procedures, performed daily, while the chance of working with the open approach is less frequent, sometimes occasional, for the majority of them. When facing a complication or a complex patient, the multifactorial attitude that includes not only technical skills, but also experience, team coordination, and decision making is of utmost importance for a positive result. The introduction of simulators devoted to acquiring skills in open and emergency surgery will be then a key point of a complete curriculum for in-training surgeons. Un-

fortunately, simulating open techniques is still more challenging and complex than is mimicking laparoscopic procedures, and will require a comprehensive, immersive environment with advanced navigation systems. Tracking of hand movement, already available, should be expanded to the whole field of operation. The use of a robotic console, as the one currently available, could be helpful in mimicking the hand movement in traditional techniques. It is important to mention that such a console, as a part of a surgical robot devoted to open surgery, is already available for clinical experimental use, being not so far from widespread applications.

- As repeatedly stated, technical skill is one of the many components of surgery. Daily clinical experience brings a considerable amount of stress, and clinical outcome can be influenced by this. Surgical simulation can greatly help in reducing this influence, with a less stressing approach to the operating theater, considering that the real procedure can be repeatedly simulated and pretested in a safe environment. Consequently, stress control should also be taught and learned virtually. Although measures are not always completely reliable, integrating biohumoral data of the trainees (collected by noninvasive methods) in a comprehensive evaluation system of the simulator could help each trainee and tutor to better identify the key points of the procedures and to understand and manage challenging situations.

- As previously briefly introduced, critical and unexpected situations (e.g., power failure, instrument breakdown) are critical part of procedures that are dependent on complex and integrated technology. Future classes of simulators should introduce randomly these accidents in their simulated procedures, in order to stimulate the creative component and the quick decisionism that have always been components of surgeons' background.

- Integrating the last concept, it is evident that group working is also a part of surgery: While introducing robotic assistants, camera holders, circulating and scrub nurses in daily practice, future simulation developers should enhance the already existing possibility to change tools, positions, etc., creating a more realistic integration with the OR environment.

Which other fields will be explored by surgery in the future? Electronics, robotics, and information technology have transformed the growth of science from linear to exponential. In the next few years, we will see many new treatments made possible by miniaturization of surgical components, such as smart materials and microrobots. The role of surgeons in a near future will be to not only eradicate, modify, or replace organs macroscopically, but also to downscale their effect on the human body at a cellular level. While simulation brands are working to reproduce codified procedures, new techniques and approach philosophies are continuously developed, more and more of them requiring an integrated, multicompetent, highly qualified team. In this field, the growth of endoluminal therapies is a typical example. The future challenges for scientist, engineers, and educators are then composed of several aspects:

- Continuing the current line of development, solving today unresolved issues through technological solutions and clearly defining the real utility of different class of simulators.
- Enhancing educational opportunities and developing training and assessment methods, with standardized, objective, criterion-based evaluation.
- Giving a consistent demonstration of transfer of skills to the operating room, with a linear relation to the improvement of the surgical performance.
- Achieving a consistent reduction of the training time, thus reducing residency length and, more important, the learning curve for new techniques.

How can we train new surgeons for new surgery, and more efficient surgeons for the old surgery? As illustrated, the burdening of knowledge of new ideas and procedures is dramatically quick, while consensus on guidelines and validation studies are mostly time-consuming and never fast enough. These considerations demonstrate that we will never be allowed to reach a static gold standard, an immutable holy grail, a dogmatic statement to define surgical simulation goals and to award the best VR simulators. Certainly, minimal requirements, efficacy, and many other aspects must be pointed out and standardized, but we must be aware that future simulators will be a component of an ongoing dynamic process, with continuous modification of surgical environment, trainees' attitude, and standards of care. The adventure has just begun.

References

Aalbakke L, Adamsen A, Kruse A (2000) Performance of a colonoscopy simulator: experience from a hands-on endoscopy course. Endoscopy 32:898–900

Adamsen S et al (2005) A comparative study of skills in virtual laparoscopy and endoscopy. Surg Endosc 19:229–234

Aggarwal R, Moorthy K, Darzi A (2004) Laparoscopic skills training and assessment. Br J Surg 91:1549–1558

Aggarwal R, Darzi A (2005) Organising a surgical skills centre. Minim Invasive Ther Allied Technol 14:275–279

Aggarwal R et al (2006) A competency-based virtual reality training curriculum for the acquisition of laparoscopic psychomotor skill. Am J Surg 191:128–111

Ahlberg G, Heikkinen T, Iselius L (2002) Does training in a virtual reality simulator improve surgical performance? Surg Endosc 16:126–129

Andreatta PB et al (2006) Laparoscopic skills are improved with LapMentor training: results of a randomized, double-blinded study. Ann Surg 243:854–860

Ayodeji ID, Schijven MP, Jakimowicz JJ (2006) Determination of face validity for the Simbionix LAP mentor virtual reality training module. Stud Health Technol Inform 119:28–30

Bergamaschi R (2000) [Farewell to see one, do one, teach one?]. TidsskrNor Laegeforen 121:2798

Blake RL, Hosokawa MC, Riley SL (2000) Student performances on step 1 and step 2 of the United States Medical Licensing. Examination following implementation of a problem-based learning curriculum. Acad Med 75:66–70

Bridges M, Diamond DL (1999) The financial impact of teaching surgical residents in the operating room. Am J Surg 177:28–32

Broe D et al (2004) Construct validation of a novel hybrid surgical simulator. Surg Endosc 20:1432–2218

Carter FJ et al (2003) Validation of a virtual reality colonoscopy simulator using subjects of differing experience (proceedings), in 1st European Endoscopic Surgical Week and 11th EAES Congress. Glasgow, UK

Carter FJ, Schijven M, Aggarwal R, Grantcharov T, Francis NK, Hanna GB, Jakimowicz JJ (2005) Consensus guidelines for validation of virtual reality surgical simulators. Surg Endosc 19:1523–1532

Chitwood WR Jr, Nifong LW, Chapman WH et al (2001) Robotic surgical training in an academic institution. Ann Surg 234:475–486

Cosman PH, Cregan PC, Martin CJ, Cartmill JA (2002) Virtual reality simulators: current status in acquisition and assessment of surgical skills. ANZ J Surg 72:30–34

Cuschieri A, Francis SN, Crosby J, Hanna GB (2001) What do master surgeons think of surgical competence and revalidation? Am J Surg 182:110–116

Custers EJFM, Regehr G, McCulloch W, Peniston C, Reznick R (1999) The effects of modeling on learning a simple surgical procedure: see one, do one or see many, do one? Adv Health Sci Educ 4:123–143

Dankelman J, Wentink M, Stassen HG (2003) Human reliability and training in minimally invasive surgery. Minim Invasive Ther Allied Technol 12:129–135

Dankelman J, Chmarra MK, Vedaasdonk EGG, Stassen LPS, Grimbergen CA (2005) Fundamental aspects of learning minimally invasive surgical skills. A review. Minim Invasive Ther Allied Technol 14:247–256

Dankelman J, Di Lorenzo N (2005) Surgical training and simulation. Minim Invasive Ther Allied Technol 14:211–213

Datta VK et al (2002) The PreOp flexible sigmoidoscopy trainer. Validation and early evaluation of a virtual reality based system. Surg Endosc 16:1459–1463

Dawson SL (2002) A critical approach to medical simulation. Bull Am Coll Surg 87:12–18

De Maria EJ, McBride CL, Broderick TJ, Kaplan BJ (2005) Night call does not impair learning of laparoscopic skills. Surg Innov 12:145–149

Deshmukh P, Carter FJ, Jayasekera BAS (2006) Face validation of a virtual reality gastroscopy simulator. Surg Endosc 20: S59)

Di Lorenzo N, Gaspari AL (2003) Virtual patient: a new option for surgical education. Business briefing publication – Global Health Care, pp 1–4

Duffy AJ et al (2003) Construct validity for the LapSim laparoscopic surgical simulator. Surg Endosc 17(Suppl 1):S230

Enochson L et al (2004) Visuospatial skills and computer game experience influence the performance of virtual endoscopy. J Gastrointest Surg 8:874–880

Eversbusch A, Grantcharov TP (2004) Learning curves and impact of psychomotor training on performance in simulated colonoscopy: a randomized trial using a virtual reality endoscopy trainer. Surg Endosc 18:1514–1518

Eriksen JR, Grantcharov TP (2005) Objective assessment of laparoscopic skills using a virtual reality simulator. Surg Endosc 19:1216–1219

Fanelli RD et al (2003) Initial experience using an endoscopic simulator to train residents in flexible endoscopy in a community medical center-based residency program. Flexible diagnostic and therapeutic endoscopy (proceedings, P233), in SAGES meeting, Los Angeles

Fellinger EF (2006) et al Complex laparoscopic task performance on two new computer-based skills training devices. Surg Endosc 20:S336

Ferlitsch A et al (2002) Evaluation of a virtual endoscopy simulator for training in gastrointestinal endoscopy. Endoscopy 34:698–702

Fried GM, Derossis AM, Bothwell J, Sigman HH (1999) Comparison of laparoscopic performance in vivo with performance measured in a laparoscopic simulator. Surg Endosc 13:1077–1081

Gallagher HJ, Allan JD, Tolley DA (2001) Spatial awareness in urologists: are they different? BJU Int 88:666–670

Gallagher AG et al (2001) Objective psychomotor skills assessment of experienced, junior and novice laparoscopists with virtual reality. World J Surg 25:1478–1483

Gallagher AG, Satava RM (2002) Virtual reality as a metric for the assessment of laparoscopic psychomotor skills: learning curves and reliability measures. Surg Endosc 16:1746–1752

Gallagher AG, Lederman AB, McGlade K, Satava RM, Smith CD (2004) Discriminative validity of the minimally invasive surgical trainer in virtual reality (MIST-VR) using criteria levels based on expert performance. Surg Endosc 18:660–665

Gallagher AG, Ritter EM, Champion H (2205) Virtual reality simulation for the operating room: proficiency-based training as a paradigm shift in surgical skills training. Ann Surg 241:364–372

Garuda S et al (2002) Efficacy of a computer-assisted endoscopic simulator in training residents in flexible endoscopy [poster], in ACG 2002 (proceedings). Seattle

Goodell KH, Cao CG, Schwaitzberg SD (2006) Effects of cognitive distraction on performance of laparoscopic surgical tasks. J Laparoendosc Adv Surg Tech A 16:94–98

Gorman PJ, Meier AH, Krummel TM (1999) Simulation and virtual reality in surgical education: real or unreal? Arch Surg 134:1203–1208

Gorman PJ, Meier AH, Krummel TM (2000) Computer-assisted training and learning in surgery. Comp Aid Surg 5:120–130

Gorman PJ, Meier AH, Rawn C, Krummel TM (2000) The future of medical education is no longer blood and guts, it is bits and bytes. Am J Surg 180:353–356

Grantcharov TP, Rosemberg J, Pahle E (2001) Virtual reality computer simulation: an objective method for evaluation of laparoscopic surgical skills. Surg Endosc 15:242–244

Grantcharov TP et al (2003) Learning curves and impact of previous operative experience on performing on a virtual reality simulator to test laparoscopic surgical skills. Am J Surg 185:146–149

Grantcharov TP et al (2204) Randomized clinical trail of virtual reality simulation for laparoscopic skills training. Br J Surg 91:146–150

Hackethal A, Immenroth M, Burger T (2006) Evaluation of target scores and benchmarks for the traversal task scenario of the Minimally Invasive Surgical Trainer – Virtual Reality (MIST-VR) laparoscopy simulator. Surg Endosc 20:645–650

Haluck RS, Marshall RL, Krummel TM, Melkonian MG (2001) Are surgery training programs ready for virtual reality? A survey of program directors in general surgery. J Am Coll Surg 193:660–665

Haluck RS, Krummel TM (2000) Computers and virtual reality for surgical education in the 21st century. Arch Surg 135:786–792

Haluck RS (2005) Design consideration for computer-based surgical simulators. Minim Invasive Ther Allied Technol 14:235–243

Halvorsen FH, Elle OJ, Fosse E (2005) Simulators in surgery. Minim Invasive Ther Allied Technol 14:214–223

Hance J et al (2004) Evaluation of a laparoscopic video trainer with built in measures of performance, in 13th SLS meeting and EndoExpo. New York

Hyltander A, Liljegren E, Rhondin PH, Lönroth H (2002) The transfer of basic skills learned in a laparoscopic simulator to the operating room. Surg Endosc 16:1324–1328

Immersion College of London. Publications of Professor Sir Ara Darzi. http://immersion.com/medical/products/hysteroscopy/case_studies.php

Issenberg SB, McGeghie WC, Hart IR et al (1999) Simulation technology for health care professional skills training and assessment. JAMA 282:861–867

Jacobs J, Caudell TP, Wilks D et al (2003) Integration of advanced technologies to enhance experiential problem-based learning over distance: Project TOUCH. Anat Rec (New Anat) 270B:16–22

Kaufmann CR (2001) Computers in surgical education and the operating room. Ann Chir Gynaecol 90:141–143

Kaufman DM, Bell W (1997) Teaching and assessing clinical skills using virtual reality. Morgan KS et al (eds.) Medicine Meets Virtual Reality. IOS, Amsterdam, pp 467–472

Kavic MS (2000) Robotics, technology, and the future of surgery. SLS 4:277–279

Kim CA, Smith CD (1999) Manual vs robotically assisted laparoscopic surgery in the performance of basic manipulation and suturing tasks. Surg Endosc 13:723

Kneebone RL, Scott W, Darzi A, Horrocks M (2004) Simulation and clinical practice: strengthening the relationship. Med Educ 38:1095–1102

Kohn LT, Corrigan JM, Donaldson MS (2000) (eds.) To err is human: building a safer health system. Committee on Quality of Health Care in America, Institute of Medicine. National Academy Press, Washington, D.C.

Korndorffer JR Jr, Stefanidis D, Scott DJ (2006) Laparoscopic skills laboratories: current assessment and a call for resident training standards. Am J Surg 2006 191:17–22

Kunst E, Rodel S, Moll F, van den Berg C, Teijink J, van Herwaarden J, van der Palen J, Geelkerken R (2006) Towards a VR trainer for EVAR treatment. Stud Health Technol Inform 119:279–281

Lange T, Indelicato DJ, Rosen JM (2000) Virtual reality in surgical training. Surg Oncol Clin N Am 9:61–79

McClusky DAM, Van Sickle K, Gallagher AG (2004) Relationship between motion analysis, time, accuracy and errors during performance of a laparoscopic suturing task on an augmented reality simulator [proceedings], in 12th EAES Congress, Barcelona

McDougall EM et al (2006) Construct validity testing of a laparoscopic surgical simulator. J Am Coll Surg 202:779–787

McNatt SS, Smith SGT (2001) A computer-based laparoscopic skills assessment device differentiates experienced from novice surgeons. Surg Endosc 15:1085–1089

Madan AK, Frantzides CT, Tebbit C, Quiros RM (2005) Participants' opinions of laparoscopic training devices after a basic laparoscopic training course. Am J Surg 189:758–761

Madan AK, Frantzides CT, Sasso LM (2005) Laparoscopic baseline ability assessment by virtual reality. Journal of Laparoscopic and Advanced Surgical Techniques 15:13–17

Mahmood T, Darzi A (2003) A study to validate the colonoscopy simulator: it is usefully discriminatory for more than one measurable outcome. Surg Endosc 17:1583–1589

Maithel S et al (2006) Construct and face validity of MIST-VR, Endotower and CELTS. Surg Endosc 20:104–112

Martin JA, Regehr G, Reznick R, Macrae H, Murnahan J, Hutchinson C, Brown M (1997) Objective structured assessment of technical skill (OSATS) for surgical residents. Br J Surg 84:273–278

Matern U, Koneczny S, Tedeus M, Dietz K, Buess G (2005) Ergonomic testing of two different types of handles via virtual reality simulation. Surg Endosc 19:1147–1150

Moorthy K et al (2004) Validity and reliability of a virtual reality upper gastrointestinal simulator and cross validation using structured assessment of individual performance with video playback. Surg Endosc 28:328–333

Munz Y, Kumar D, Moorthy S et al (2004) Laparoscopic virtual reality and box trainers: is one superior to the other? Surg Endosc 18:485–494

Mutter D, Rubino F, Temporal MSG, Marescaux J (2005) Surgical education and Internet-based simulation: The World Virtual University. Minim Invasive Ther Allied Technol 14:267–274

Ost D et al (2001) Assessment of a bronchoscopy simulator. Am J Respir Crit Care Med 164:2248–2255

Ota D, Loftin B, Saito T, Lea R, Keller J (1995) Virtual Reality in Surgical Education. Comput Biol Med 25:127–137

Patel AD, Gallagher AG, Nicholson WJ, Cates CU (2006) Learning curves and reliability measures for virtual reality simulation in the performance assessment of carotid angiography. J Am Coll Cardiol 47:1796–1802

Rasmussen R (1983) Skills, rules and knowledge; signals, signs and symbols, and other distinctions in human performance models. IEEE Trans. Systems Man Cybernetics 13:257–266

Reich O, Noll M, Gratzke C, Bachmann A, Waidelich R, Seitz M, Schlenker B, Baumgartner R, Hofstetter A, Stief CG (2006) High-level virtual reality simulator for endourologic procedures of lower urinary tract. Urology 67:1144–1148

Ritter EM et al (2005) Objective psychomotor skills assessment of experienced and novice flexible endoscopists with a virtual reality simulator. J Gastrointest Surg 7:871–878

Ritter EM, Bowyer MW (2005) Simulation for trauma and combat casualty care. Minim Invasive Ther Allied Technol 14:224–234

Rosenthal R, Gantert WA, Scheidegger D, Oertli D (2006) Can skills assessment on a virtual reality trainer predict a surgical trainee's talent in laparoscopic surgery? Surg Endosc 20:1286–1290

Rovetta L (2000) A computer assisted surgery with 3D robot models and visualisation of the telesurgical action Stud Health Technol Inform 70:292–294

Rovetta A, Bejczy AK, Sala R (1997) Telerobotic surgery: applications on human patients and training with virtual reality. Stud Health Technol Inform 39:508–517

Rowe R, Cohen R (2000) Virtual reality bronchoscopy simulator [proceedings], in ASA annual meeting, 2000

Rowe R, Cohen RA (2002) An evaluation of a virtual reality airway simulator. Anesth Analg 95:62–66

Sanders AJ, Luursema JM, Warntjes P, Mastboom WJ, Geelkerken RH, Klaase JM, Rodel SG, ten Cate Hoedemaker HO, Kommers PA, Verwey WB, Kunst EE (2006) Validation of open-surgery VR trainer. Stud Health Technol Inform 119:473–476

Satava RM (2002) Disruptive vision: moral and ethical challenges from advanced technology and issues for the new generation of surgeons. Surg Endosc 16:1403–1408

Satava RM (1995) Medical applications of virtual reality. J Med Syst 19275–280

Satava RM, Gallagher AG, Pellegrini CA (2003) Surgical competence and surgical proficiency: definitions, taxonomy, and metrics. J Am Coll Surg 196:933–937

Satava RM (2005) Identification and reduction of surgical error using simulation: an overview. Minim Invasive Ther Allied Technol 14:257–261

Schijven M, Jakimowicz J (2003) Virtual reality surgical laparoscopic simulators: how to choose. Surgic Endosc 17:1943–1950

Schijven M, Jakimowicz J (2005) Validation of virtual reality simulators: key to the successful integration of a novel teaching technology into minimal access surgery. Minim Invasive Ther Allied Technol 14:244–246

Seymour NE, Gallagher AG, Roman SA, O'Brien MK, Bansal VK, Anderson DK, Satava RM (2002) Virtual reality training improves operating room performance: results of a randomized, double-blinded study. Ann Surg 236:458–464

Seymour NE (2005) Integratine simulation into a busy residency program. Minim Invasive Ther Allied Technol 14:280–286

Sloan DA, Donnelly MB, Schwartz RW, Strodel WE (1995) The Objective Structured Clinical Examination: the new gold standard for evaluating postgraduate clinical performance. Ann Surg 222:735–742

Scott DJ, Bergen PC, Rege RV, Laycock R, Tesfay ST, Valentine RJ, Euhus DM, Jeyarajah DR, Thompson WM, Jones DB (2000) Laparoscopic training on bench models: better and more cost effective than operating room experience. J Am Coll Surg 191:272–283

Sedlack RE, Kolars JC (2003) Validation of a computer-based colonoscopy simulator. Gastrointest Endosc 57:214–218

Sedlack RE, Kolars JC (2004) Computer simulator training enhances the competency of gastroenterology fellows at colonoscopy: results of a pilot study. Am J Gastroenterol 99:33–37

Seymour NE et al (2002) Virtual reality improves operating room performance: results of a randomized, double-blind study. Ann Surg 236:458–463

Seymour NE (2005) Integrating simulation into a busy residency program. Minim Invasive Ther Allied Technol 14:280–286

Sickle KR van et al (2005) Construct validation of the ProMis simulator using a novel laparoscopic suturing task. Surg Endosc 19:1227–1231

Stefanidis D, Haluck R, Pham T, Dunne JB, Reinke T, Markley S, Korndorffer JR Jr, Arellano P, Jones DB, Scott DJ (2006) Construct and face validity and task workload for laparoscopic camera navigation: virtual reality versus videotrainer systems at the SAGES Learning Center. Surg Endosc doi:10.1007/s00464-006-9112-9

Stefanidis D, Korndorffer JR Jr, Black FW, Dunne JB, Sierra R, Touchard CL, Rice DA, Markert RJ, Kastl PR, Scott DJ (2006) Psychomotor testing predicts rate of skill acquisition for proficiency-based laparoscopic skills training. Surgery 140:252–262

Stefanidis D, Korndorffer JR Jr, Sierra R, Touchard C, Dunne JB, Scott DJ (2005) Skill retention following proficiency-based laparoscopic simulator training. Surgery 138:165–170

Taffinder NJ et al (1998) An objective assessment of surgeons' psychomotor skills: validation of the MIST-VR laparoscopic simulator. Br J Surg 85(Suppl 1):75

Takiguchi S, Sekimoto M, Yasui M, Miyata H, Fujiwara Y, Yasuda T, Yano M, Monden M (2005) Cyber visual training as a new method for the mastery of endoscopic surgery. Surg Endosc 19:1204–10

Thomas-Gibson S, Vance ME, Saunders BP (2003) Can a colonoscopy computer simulator differentiate between a novice and expert? [Abstract]. Gut 52(Suppl 1):A73

Torkington J, Smith SG, Rees B, Darzi A (2001) The role of the basic surgical skills course in the acquisition and retention of laparoscopic skill. Surg Endosc 15:1071–1075

Uchal M, Tjugum J, Martinsen E, Qiu X, Bergamaschi R (2005) The impact of sleep deprivation on product quality and procedure effectiveness in a laparoscopic physical simulator: a randomized controlled trial. Am J Surg 189:753–757

Van Sickle KR, Ritter EM, McClusky DA III, Lederman A, Baghai M, Gallagher AG, Smith CD (2006) Attempted establishment of proficiency levels for laparoscopic performance on a national scale using simulation: the results from the 2004 SAGES Minimally Invasive Surgical Trainer-Virtual Reality (MIST-VR) learning center study. Surg Endosc 21:5–10

Varley RJ, Goodall JE, Bingener J (2006) Can proficiency benchmarks be established using the endoscopic simulator. Surg Endosc 20:S342

Verdaasdonk EG, Stassen LP, Monteny LJ, Dankelman J (2006) Validation of a new basic virtual reality simulator for training of basic endoscopic skills: the SIMENDO. Surg Endosc 20:511–518

Yousfi MM et al (2002) Flexible sigmoidoscopy: assessing endoscopic skills using a computer-based simulator [proceedings], in ACG meeting, 2002. Seattle

Waseda M, Inaki N, Mailander L, Buess GF (2005) An innovative trainer for surgical procedures using animal organs. Minim Invasive Ther Allied Technol 14:262–266

Wentink M, Stassen LPS, Alwayn I, Hosman RJAW, Stassen HG (2003) Rasmussen's model of human behaviour in laparoscopy training. Surgic Endosc 17:1241–1246

The Medical Informatics Challenge in Surgery

8

J. Sutherland and Timothy Ganous

This chapter focuses on the unique challenge that the operating room represents for medical information technologies developers. It also addresses the need to focus future development of information technologies in a manner consistent with experiences of other non-medical industries.

8.1 The Perioperative Environment

The perioperative environment is one of the most technologically advanced areas of the modern health care enterprise. From the anesthesia machine to the physiologic monitors to advanced imaging devices, the use of computer technology in the operating room now collects and displays thousands of data points per hour. It would be reasonably sound to make the claim that the computing power that resides in the typical operating room today could form the basis of a small, dedicated supercomputing cluster found in most academic computer science departments. Very rarely, however, is there the intent or capability of integrating this computing power or the information systems that medical devices host in order to make the perioperative process more efficient and patient care more effective.

The barriers to integration have been well documented and discussed by many frustrated clinicians [38]. This common concern has spawned little commitment in the health care industry, surgery in particular, in the direction of integration and interoperability. Medical device manufacturers continue to produce valuable breakthrough technologies that can successfully fit into clinical practice models as stand-alone components. When integration is offered, it is usually in the form of proprietary add-ins or suites of instrumentation. Other than being network capable and accessible with unique intranet protocol addressing, very little work has been forthcoming in the area of common data structures, machine-to-machine languages, and machine-to-hospital information data exchange schema that would foster true interoperability of information. However, common industry data protocols

such as HL7 [18], which were created for the exchange of medical information between providers, payers, and regulators, has highlighted the glaring lack of interoperability of technologies in most clinical settings, including surgery.

The practice models currently utilized in surgery today were designed and implemented decades before the information technologies we rely on today were envisioned. The fact that these models survive in spite of the explosion of technology embedded in surgery is atypical of evolution of information technology in almost every other industry. The key feature of coordination in most processes associated with surgery continues to be human-to-human communication. That is why telephone, fax, and e-mail continue to have such prominence in the surgical suite. It is particularly troubling that the ever-increasing complexity of technology and clinical protocols in surgery will continue to be managed by perioperative staff performing job descriptions that have not changed except for the lengthening list of technology implementations, patient care responsibilities, and regulatory requirements.

The culture of surgery has also been slow in transforming along with the technology in its midst. In a national surgical conference held in Baltimore, Maryland, in 2002 it was noted by the keynote speaker, Dr. Bruce Jarrell, that surgery today could be characterized in the following manner:

- Teamwork is fragmented.
- Communications are by voice and grease board.
- A significant amount of energy goes into making it function rather than patient care.
- Surgeon personalities are a strong factor in its operation.
- The workload is highly variable but has high peaks.
- The complexity is high.
- Time is wasted. Someone in the operating room is always looking for some critical thing while the patient and surgeon wait.
- Information systems are used to a limited degree.

The issues, as identified by Dr. Jarrell, are classic production problems experienced in most other industries, including manufacturing, finance, and transportation among many others, and were early targets of technology-based solutions. A hospital-based surgical unit's exposure to technology-based solutions developed by other industries often occurs in the form of contracted relationships with business partners, a predominant example being automating supply chain processes. In this case, operating room staffs are frequently not the sponsors of the new technology solutions but are invited users of the solutions.

What is found in most modern surgical suites are surgical and anesthesiology information systems. Both perform scheduling, coordination of preoperative processes, and case management and medical coding functions. Anesthesia systems typically go beyond these basic functions and utilize data extracted from connected monitoring and other medical devices to populate a medical encounter record, usually based on proprietary solutions. These systems are often justified based on revenue capture although they have significant patient safety and outcome implications.

8.1.1 Why Adapt Solutions from Other Industries?

The pace of change and number of events that need monitoring in a high-velocity trauma center or large surgery facility with dozens of operating rooms make manual analysis and control of daily operations difficult, painful, and inefficient. Methods are needed to automate standard protocols, to monitor execution of processes, and to alert staff about required interventions. A useful metaphor for solving these problems is the introduction of the autopilot in the aircraft industry. Initially, autopilots were simple devices that kept the aircraft level and on course while the crew could pay attention to higher-level tasks. As flying became faster and more risky in aerial combat, terrain-following radar was introduced to drive an autopilot that would fly a fighter aircraft at the speed of sound at 500 ft in mountainous terrain at night. These systems have now evolved to full control of takeoff and landing of commercial airliners. The first Boeing test flights of new aircraft are done by autopilots to avoid risking the lives of crewmembers.

An interesting aspect of autopilots is that they operate by feedback mechanisms that cause small corrections back on course, so that large corrections are never needed. This is critical in health care where early, small interventions in patient treatment can often easily avoid disastrous outcomes. Interventions that are too late and require large corrections can be damaging and even fatal. An autopilot is needed to guide process execution for routine health care events, and warning lights and alarms need to be available just as they are

for an aircraft pilot when an engine is overheating or a collision is immanent. Health care is in great need of an air traffic control system that assures operating rooms are ready, staff and equipment are in place, the patient is properly staged and prepped through the process, and beds and follow-up treatment are available when the patient clears the operating room.

As concerns about patient safety have grown, the health care sector has looked to other industries that have confronted similar challenges, in particular the airline industry. This industry learned long ago that information and clear communication are critical to the safe navigation of an airplane. To perform their jobs well and guide their planes safely to their destinations, pilots must communicate with the air traffic controller concerning their destinations and current circumstances (e.g., mechanical or other problems), their flight plans, and environmental factors (e.g., weather conditions) that could necessitate a change in course. Information must also pass seamlessly from one controller to another to ensure a safe and smooth journey for planes flying long distances; provide notification of airport delays or closures due to weather conditions; and enable rapid alert and response to an extenuating circumstance, such as a terrorist attack.

Institute of Medicine (US) Committee on Quality
of Health Care in America [19]

In a perioperative setting, hundreds of patients and staff may be flowing through dozens of operating rooms on a daily basis in a single facility. A third of the patients are unscheduled and identified only on the day of surgery. The resulting chaos can be overwhelming, even with some form of electronic health record (EHR) system (currently available in 12% of hospital systems [38]). Orchestration of behavior between information systems is people and paper based. Available automated systems are often dedicated to isolated operations or departments with no automated means to communicate with one other. The limitations of this environment provide great opportunity for process improvement efforts. A 30% improvement can be routinely achieved in almost any targeted area and 100% improvements are possible [34].

8.2 Radical Improvement in Quality of Patient Care is Possible

Enhanced automation and integration to avoid oversights, mistakes, and medical errors are only the tip of the iceberg in improvement possibilities for health care. Radical improvement in the overall quality of care is possible not only by reducing the incidence of medical errors, but also by deeply reinventing existing health care processes.

Important areas for business process redesign related to the success of current medical practices entails research of new clinical protocols and design of disease management systems. Business process integration offers a promising solution for rapid adoption of new treatments in practice by promoting new techniques through automated alerts and recommendations, while reducing negative side effects by displaying warnings and recent analyses of outcomes.

For example, it currently takes an average of 17 years for evidence-based medicine to be integrated into clinical practice [5], and research shows that physicians incorporate the latest medical evidence into treatment only about 50% of the time.

Our results indicate that, on average, Americans receive about half of recommended medical care processes. Although this point estimate of the size of the quality problem may continue to be debated, the gap between what we know works and what is done is substantial enough to warrant attention. These deficits, which pose serious threats to the health and well-being of the US public, persist despite initiatives by both the federal government and private health care delivery systems to improve care.
S. Marsland and I. Buchan [24]

Opportunities for unobtrusively automating the introduction, suggestion, or recommendation of the latest evidence-based medical practice into clinical processes could generate a revolutionary improvement in patient outcomes. The impact of monitoring and managing small increments of clinical behavior can have enormous consequences. A recent study [31] showed that

inpatient medication error is the fourth leading cause of death in the United States (113,000 deaths), with nosocomial infections not far behind (90,000 deaths). Inpatient surgery and postoperative care appear to significantly contribute to adverse events. An analysis of 15,000 nonpsychiatric hospital discharges revealed that 66% of adverse events were found related to surgery [7]. For example, failure to give antibiotics within 2 h before surgery doubles the postoperative deep wound and organ space infection rate, compounding medical error with nosocomial infection (Fig. 8.1). Automated monitoring and alerting on this relatively simple event generates a significant improvement in care [20].

Automated monitoring of order entry and medication administration is easily implemented with new information systems coming on line. Even with older systems, for example, it is currently possible with systems in place at the University of Maryland Medical Center (UMMC) to monitor order status of a medication and to generate an automated query to a care provider prior to patient surgery to confirm proper antibiotic delivery.

8.3   Toward a Solution: Adaptive Process Control

Wireless communication devices, context-aware applications, and adaptive workflow engines can help overcome problems identified by Operating Room of the Future experts. Health care processes require coordinating not only many concurrent administra-

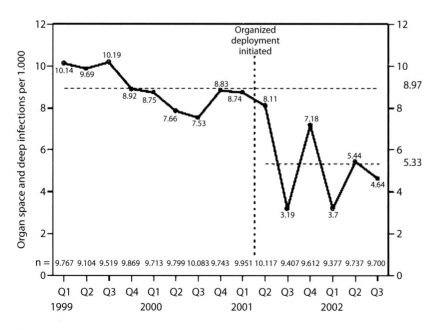

Fig. 8.1 Postoperative deep wound and organ space infection rates per 1,000 elective surgical cases [19]

tive processes, but also clinical events and the patient scenario within a health care enterprise that can span many departments and extended periods. In addition, health care workflows are notably dynamic because of regular upgrade of treatment protocols and unexpected changes in patient status or response to treatment [3].

It is important to note that workflow systems implemented in most industrial settings are inappropriate for health care. For example, ERP systems are increasingly adopting standards-based workflow engines to control process flow. These systems are typically designed to control "predictive processes". implying that the steps of the process are highly predictable in advance.

Health care workflows can be highly *unpredictable* due to organizational or medical complexity. What is most interesting and important is what goes wrong and how the quickly the system can adapt to unexpected events [10]. At UMMC, for example, a third of the surgeries are unanticipated and enter the process at unpredictable times during the day. These unexpected behaviors have unpredictable implications for the well-understood and planned activities. A highly adaptive system is needed to help control this "empirical process." In the chemical industry where process research is a core competency, applying a "predictive process" system to control an "empirical process" has caused many plant explosions [26]. In health care, this same mistake will also increase morbidity and mortality.

Complex adaptive system theory has been applied to analysis of information systems in health care and other industries [33]. All that follows should be interpreted with the understanding that a health care enterprise is viewed as a complex adaptive system [23, 39].

8.4   Context-Aware Workflow as Autopilot

The effective use of adaptive workflow engines in the health care enterprise can be thought of as an autopilot. A simple autopilot does not fly the plane, and it does not perform the tasks of aircraft subsystems. It monitors and observes that a process is veering off an established course. It alerts the pilot to unusual events and makes minor adjustments in trajectory by gently tweaking subsystems to push the aircraft toward level flight on a predetermined heading. In this way, the autopilot prevents major errors by handling multiple small errors and correcting them. More advanced autopilots use terrain following radar and other subsystems to automatically fly the plane. However, even then, they rely on a hierarchy of subsystems to actually execute flight.

For example, in designing a robotic system like the DARPA Trauma Pod, which is planned to autonomously perform surgery on the battlefield, a workflow engine will not do the surgery. It will check that the

Trauma Pod is ready for surgery, handle the logistic aspects of assuring supplies and instruments are available, cleanup after robotic surgery is complete, restock, sanitize, and prepare for the next surgery. In addition, it will assure no sponges are left inside the patient, using Radio Frequency IDentification (RFID) technology. When it sees exceptions, it will alert hierarchical subsystems or external systems to take appropriate action. This approach, which MIT Prof. Rodney Brooks calls a "subsumption" architecture, is a way to take a large collection of dumb subsystems and orchestrate them to exhibit intelligent behavior in robotic design [8]. The same approach can be taken to monitor heterogeneous distributed systems in a health care enterprise, which are "dumb" in the sense they cannot communicate well with one another or adjust well to one another. A higher-level workflow engine operating like an autopilot can alert subsystems or clinicians to perform adjustments to patient processes before major problems occur. Hence, in this manner, a large collection of dumb subsystems can be made to appear "smart."

An adaptive workflow engine can be used to orchestrate the behavior of the many disparate health care systems in a surgery center through direct integration via Web services, HL7 standards-based messaging, a hybrid solution, or proprietary adaptors [32]. The ability to "capture" the function of legacy components in an enterprise is a standard complex adaptive systems strategy and the basis for introduction of intelligent agents into advanced software systems [4].

Another important aspect of an autopilot is total situational awareness of what is happening with subsystems and using that awareness to unobtrusively alter aircraft behavior. The pilot of an aircraft wants an autopilot to do its task so well that its operations are transparent. In order to promote user adoption of new clinical processes in a health care enterprise, the workflow engine must be transparent to routine operations and only become visible when a critical event occurs. The introduction of RFID technology for capture of critical data on patients, staff, instruments, and supplies helps to make this possible.

8.5   Stealth Mode: Automated Data Collection

A stealth mode of data collection is needed to introduce new technology without disrupting current manual processes. By stealth mode, we mean automated collection of data that is normally observed, yet irregularly captured because of lack of time and tedious manual data entry procedures. It is essential data for managing operations that is irregularly registered in a high-stress environment, leading to erroneous perceptions that generate to suboptimal organizational response.

RFID technology can automatically monitor flow of patients, staff, supplies, and equipment. Baseline data can be captured for critical process points, bottlenecks identified, and process improvement plans developed. Monitoring critical events and evoking selective orchestration of behavior is required across multiple health care information systems and care providers that move a patient through the perioperative system with dozens of points of clinical and administrative interaction.

Passively monitoring operations with RFID technology provides real-time data useful in constraint theory analyses [16], an approach that can identify bottlenecks and target selected initiatives that cause radical improvement in throughput in an enterprise in a short period. In addition, sensing systems combined with workflow engines and inferencing applications can anticipate future events, and trigger interventions that alter the course of action, potentially saving patients' lives, and certainly improving efficiency. RFID capabilities are now being integrated into 802.11 access points such that the RFID data can be seamlessly delivered to a central network or database, with transaction specific accuracy for the location of patients, staff, and hospital assets [14]. Future refinements will allow real-time determination of procedures performed by proximity of a clinicians, patient, and instruments for an appropriate period. Intelligent video can identify the nature of processes underway in an operating room.

Baseline data gathered can be used for targeting high-yield process interventions. In the initial phases, this category of process improvements targets should be implemented manually. When the manual solution demonstrates success and the return on investment (ROI) is positive, real-time process monitoring can be implemented to sustain initial gains, widely deploy the implementation within the organization, and support an ongoing process improvement methodology.

Data mining of historical information can generate new insights for process intervention. Real-time adaptation, combined with postprocess automated reflection generating new strategies for future adaptation is a powerful feedback process that can progress a system from strength to strength through continuous process improvement.

8.6 A RECIPE for Incremental Systems Evolution and Process Improvement

The health care goals of increasing revenue, reducing cost, enhancing patient care, and improving customer satisfaction are difficult to achieve due to high costs of integration of legacy systems, cultural barriers to adoption, and the intrinsically complex nature of health care

processes. Health care processes typically require deep knowledge and expertise, are highly error prone, and demand a significant requirement for cross-functional workflow [13]. These issues present many barriers to adoption of new technologies.

Research results from the Operating Room of the Future project at the University of Maryland, valuable insights from the business school and computer science departments of the University of Tilburg in the Netherlands, and feedback from the annual Future of Health Technology Summit at the Massachusetts Institute of Technology have led to the development of a process for technology introduction that maximizes probability of successful adoption by minimizing disruption of ongoing surgery operations. We call this process a RECIPE for REal-Time proCess ImProvement in health care [36].

RECIPE focuses on identifying bottlenecks in current processes that can lead to development of small incremental improvements. Most opportunities for intervention can generate 30% improvement, and 100% improvements are often achieved [34]. Strategically introducing small incremental changes into current processes can evolve over time into major institutional transformation.

The RECIPE for incremental evolution of administrative and clinical processes consists of a planning component, a testing component, and a technology component.

The planning component is the responsibility of clinical domain experts and requires:

- High-level mapping of end-to-end health care processes
- Prioritizing opportunities for operational or clinical improvements
- Detailed process mapping of selected process improvement areas
- Selection of precise mechanism for process improvements
- Establishment of research objectives and collected of data for outcomes analysis

For example, the flow sheet below shows a high level mapping of the patient visit needed to prepare for surgery. Other data collected show that some steps in this process are not completed in time or not completed at all prior to surgery, causing delays. More detailed analysis of exactly what happens at delay points allows capture of baseline data and selection of specific actions for process improvement. When a process improvement is introduced, follow-up data is compared to baseline data based on a research protocol established prior to the study. Formalized collection and analysis of research data allows validation of findings and data quality required for publication of research results (Fig. 8.2).

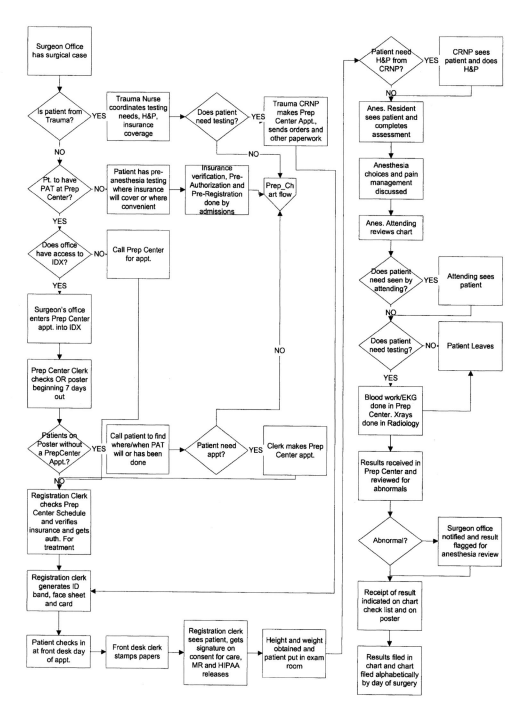

Fig. 8.2 Perioperative process map of patient preparation visit prior to surgery at the University of Maryland Medical Center data prepared under contract with Perioptimum on 24 May 2004

The testing component requires:

- Communication and validation of planned improvements with all stakeholders
- Manual introduction of the process change in a targeted area of the institution
- Data collection to document the effect of the process change
- Recommendations for automation of the process improvement

The technology component requires domain knowledge and expertise in new technologies areas. Specifically:

- RFID technologies need to be evaluated, pilot projects initiated, and data collection and monitoring strategies need to be defined.
- Workflow engines are increasingly embedded in ERP and CRM systems for specifying, automating, and updating operational protocols. This technology needs to be evaluated, selected, and fine-tuned for health care operations.
- Alerting and messaging systems need to be implemented to reach any member of the clinical or operational staff on any available device.
- Service-oriented architectures (SOAs) need to be deployed to provide cost-effective integration with enterprise and departmental systems.
- An operational database needs to be established to store protocol specifications, state of protocol executions, and essential data collected as part of a medical encounter record (MER) that is used for workflow execution.
- Dynamic real-time application generation of workflow requests for action or information is specified and implemented.
- Automated reporting is essential for real-time operations information and data mining of historical workflow data.
- Monitoring and reporting on changes in baseline data affected by incremental process improvement needs to be automatically delivered to clinical and administrative staff on a routine basis to demonstrate and maintain process improvements.

The focus of all these efforts is to bring knowledge gained in other industries into health care, such as airport logistics [15], where deployment of these techniques has placed Amsterdam Airport Schiphol in the top three airports in the world with respect to the passenger experience. Throughput can typically be enhanced in virtually all operations: inventory can be reduced through just in time delivery, quality can be enhanced, and patient satisfaction of medical products can be optimized through innovation and fine-tuning at the level of individual clients.

Boston Medical Center, the city's safety net hospital, is becoming a model of how to bring relief to the nation's beleaguered emergency rooms, reducing treatment delays and closures to ambulances when ERs are more crowded than ever. BMC emergency doctors are treating more patients than they did last year and have reduced average time in the waiting room from 60 minutes to 40 minutes. The secret lies in a radical idea for medicine, but one that has guided airport managers and restaurant hostesses for years: Keep the customers moving.

S. Allen [1]

8.7 Applying the RECIPE to Perioperative Systems Design

Perioperative systems design describes a rational approach to managing the convergent flow of patients having procedures from disparate physical and temporal starting points, through the operating room and then to such a place where future events pertaining to the patient have no further impact on operating room operations (Fig 8.3). This process for an individual patient can be envisioned as a nested set of timelines: a coarse-grained timeline beginning with the decision to perform an operation and ending when the patient definitively leaves the postoperative occurrence, and a fine-grained timeline encompassing the immediate pre-, intra-, and postoperative course. At each point, physical infrastructure and work processes affect the progress of patients along these timelines. Starting from this construct, perioperative systems design can be conceptualized, studied, and optimized like any industrial process in which many materials, actors, and processes are brought together in a coordinated workflow to achieve a designed goal. Figure 8.3 shows nested, interactive timelines around the preoperative period, the intraoperative period, and the postoperative period. Of interest, is that there are as more activities before and after surgery than during surgery.

8.8 Perioperative Systems Acceleration Tool in the Preoperative Period

In the preoperative period the Perioperative Systems Acceleration Tool (PSPAT) needs to orchestrate and monitor the following activities:
- Patient identification
- Diagnostic workup
- Incoming patient medications and allergies;
- Surgery schedule
- Determine staff readiness

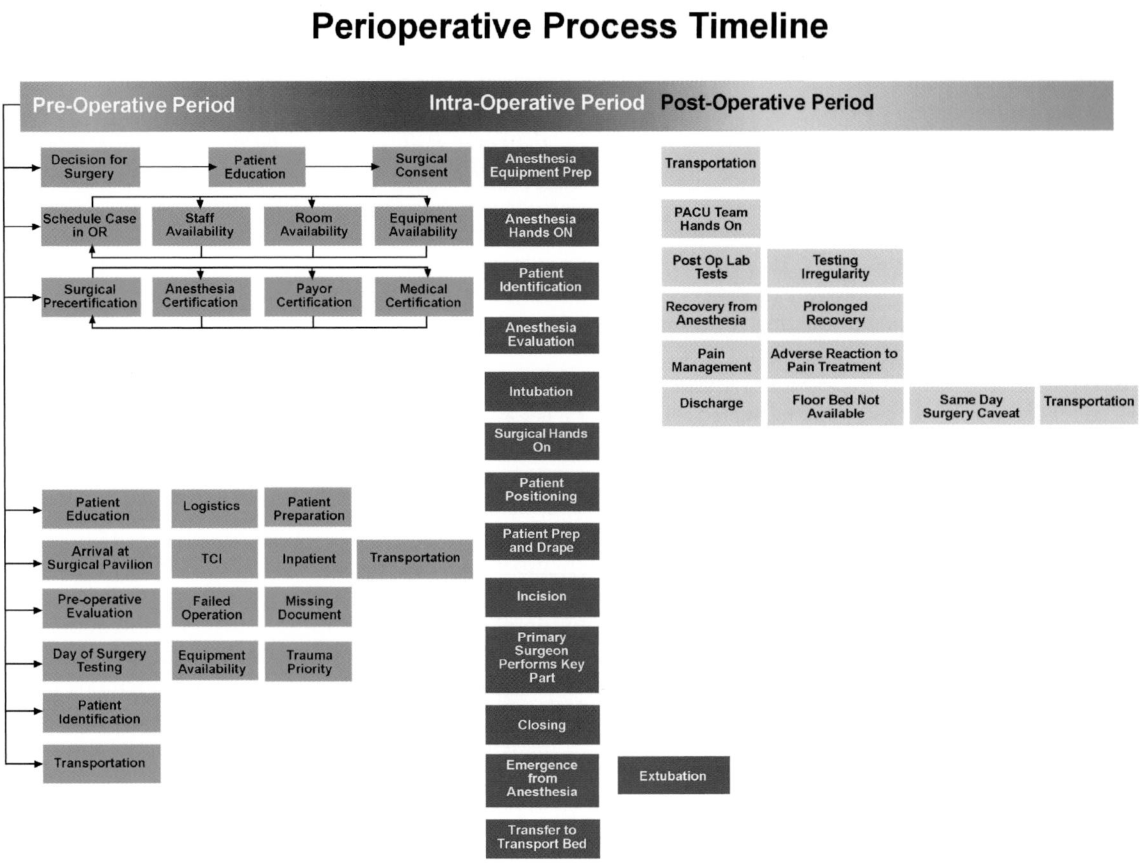

Perioperative Process Timeline

Fig. 8.3 Perioperative process timeline [30]

- Confirm operating room readiness
- Assure supplies and equipment availability
- Capture data on incoming medical record, capture vitals, inputs/outputs (I/Os), preoperative medications, tests, and scans
- Monitor patient entry into operating room
- Monitor patient readiness

The first two tasks serve to identify the patient and the corresponding diagnoses so to avoid any mistakes. For example, wrong-site surgery makes up 2% of medical error [17]. A surgery scheduling system is used to schedule patient, staff, and operating room. At UMMC, a third of surgeries each day are unscheduled; the scheduling problem is extremely difficult in a surgical setting. There are many moving parts to be coordinated and many unanticipated events.

Supplies and equipment must be prepared before surgery, and the case cart with all items needed must be in the operating room before surgery. Case cart readiness was a major problem at UMMC prior to be-

ginning this study. A substantial amount of paperwork and lab tests must be gathered an interpreted before surgery. There are many points where delays can be induced in the system. As a result, surgery start times are often late, which has major revenue and cost implications. Process mapping and monitoring of critical points can significantly increase patient throughput.

Monitoring patient entry into the operating room and patient readiness for surgery are critical to successful outcomes, particularly with respect to patient safety. Automated monitoring of positioning and timing of the patient can reduce manual data entry, increase accuracy, and provide analytical data essential to planning for process improvement. However, some important processes need to remain manual. One of the best processes has been established at the Massachusetts General Operating Room of the Future facility, where the surgeon talks with the patient just prior to anesthesia. The patient is asked, without any prompting information, why he or she is there, what procedure is to be performed, and where it is to be preformed. The patient points to the spot and the surgeon confirms it has been marked properly. The attending surgeon then asks the resident surgeon to check the medical records of the patient and confirm that everything the patient just stated is in the record. The patient is then anesthetized and brought into the operating room. Prior to start of the procedure, the attending surgeon repeats to the surgical team exactly why the patient is there and what procedure is to be accomplished. The team is asked if they agree. There is a moment of silence until every person on the team gives indication of assent before the procedure begins. This process is very much like a preflight check when operating a military or commercial aircraft. Careful attention to detailed procedures and cross checks prevents many disasters. Unfortunately, this process is not rigorously followed in most operating rooms.

8.9   PSPAT in the Intraoperative Period

Intraoperative tasks include:
- Anesthesia equipment preparation
- Anesthesia
- Patient identification
- Anesthesia evaluation
- Intubation
- Surgical hands-on
- Patient positioning
- Patient prep and drape
- Incision
- Primary surgery
- Closing
- Emergence from anesthesia
- Extubation
- Patient transport

PSPAT assumes that the anesthesiologist intubates and monitors the patient while the surgical team does the surgery. It monitors surgery start and stop times, manages schedule irregularities, assures proper inventory of supplies, instruments, and equipment, and communications externally when operating room needs arise. Patient safety is supported by patient identification and RFID technology used to check inventory and make sure no supplies are left inside the patient.

8.10   PSPAT in the Postoperative Period

Postoperative issues include:
- Patient transportation
- Patient handoff to recovery area
- Postop lab tests
- Assessing lab test irregularities
- Monitoring recovery from anesthesia
- Dealing with issues around prolonged recovery
- Pain management
- Adverse reaction to pain treatment
- Discharge

When surgery is complete, the patient is moved to a recovery area and monitored carefully. Appropriate laboratory tests are performed, and any abnormalities are assessed for further treatment. Pain is carefully managed along with any adverse reactions to the surgery, allergic responses, and postsurgery medication or treatment.

All of these issues need to be deal with by a combination of human and automated systems. At a minimum, PSPAT maintains an MER. This consists of all relevant data on patient flow through the perioperative process. It is collected, processed, evaluated, and updated by a workflow engine. The MER provides data for the discharge summary, and updates the external medical record. In addition, PSPAT may be tasked with monitoring protocols around lab tests and pain management, as well interfacing with transportation subsystems and handoff of the patient to external systems.

8.11   PSPAT at the University of Maryland Medical Center

The University of Maryland Medical System designed a PSPAT that provides an integrated workflow engine, rules engine, logistics engine, MER repository, and interface engine, coupled with extensive connectivity to all relevant external enterprise systems. PSPAT will passively monitor the location and availability of patients, staff, supplies, instruments, equipment, and operating facilities; watch the convergence of the surgery team, supplies, instruments, and equipment around the patient and intervene to assure that critical personnel and physical requirements are met in real time; and initiate alternative protocols and actions when planned perioperative schedules cannot be met or patient safety is at risk.

The basic concepts in PSPAT are information uptake from a wide variety of clinical systems; calculation of current state of clinical processing; and generating a set of reactions to current state in order to move it towards organizational goals for efficiency, safety, and improvement of patient outcomes (Fig. 8.4).

In the context of an automated operating room of the future, it is essential to wrap information technology around the surgery to support the entire perioperative

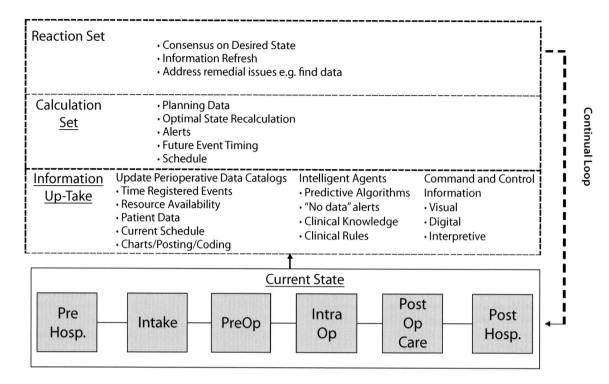

Fig. 8.4 Perioperative Systems Process Acceleration Tool (PSPAT)

process, and orchestrate behavior between heterogeneous systems that exist outside, yet support the surgical procedure, and are mandatory for patient safety and support of treatment before and after surgery. In particular, it is essential to provide a lightweight MER repository capable of managing the information input of a patient record, diagnostic and triage information, vitals and I/Os data collection, automated lab tests and patient scans, treatment plans, order sets and protocols, surgeon preference lists for supplies and equipment, Web-based visual display of patient information for external telemedicine clinicians, and reordering and restocking supplies management. Postsurgical care, discharge summaries, and externally posting of updates to the patient's medical record are essential. The medical facility picking up the patient for postsurgical care must have up to date medical information that incorporates all procedures, medications, and diagnoses, along with discharge medications and recommendations for follow-up.

PSPAT will use existing clinical and logistics systems to the maximum extent possible. For example, there is an enterprise-wide clinical repository that supports computerized physician order entry. Several equipment and supply information systems support perioperative activities. Integration with these systems allows PSPAT to use these systems as both data sources and implementation systems for adaptive process improvement.

8.12 PSPAT Components

This section provides a conceptual overview of PSPAT. In some cases technology is available and implemented. In others, selection activities are underway. Some components are in the prototype stage. All are based on available commercial products.

8.12.1 A Workflow Engine

The workflow engine is the heart of the PSPAT. It understands the steps of the perioperative system design and beats as it executes perioperative processes step by step. It pumps information and moves it through various organ systems of the PSPAT. The organ systems provide services to the workflow engine that help it execute its tasks. The key service components of the workflow engine are (1) adapters to extract information from any human or machine source of essential data; (2) a virtual information repository to store the MER, along with process definitions and key information elements required for process execution; (3) a rules engine to do intelligence processing of essential information to answer questions posed by the workflow engine as to current state; (4) an alerting and messaging system to inform or request other parts of the health care system to perform tasks, request information, or advise on completion of critical tasks; (5) a reporting system to monitor timely task completion and provide summary data for outcomes analysis; (6) a logistics subsystem to manage inventory and ordering of supplies, instruments, and equipment; and (7) a Web-based telemedicine view of all data and process states for external human interaction and observation.

Workflow engines designed to streamline, automate, and re-engineer business processes are rarely deployed in health care. Here we assess the most prevalent initiatives in this domain. For this purpose, it is important to make a distinction between workflow management systems products of the 1990s, which were monolithic in nature, and current workflow engines designed to be embedded as a software tool in a service-oriented architecture [22]. The most advanced workflow engine prototype for health care designed specifically for Web-based integration with legacy systems was Big Workflow, developed at IDX Systems in the late 1990s in collaboration with computer scientists from IBM Watson Laboratories [28, 29, 32]. Several prototypes have been developed for clinical and administrative systems using the University of Georgia METEOR Workflow Management System [3]. Strategies for using workflow technology to capture legacy systems and repurpose them for use with more current technologies are critical for health care and have been well documented [33]. Enterprise modeling for business process transformation in health care, serving as a basis for configuring medical workflow engines, has been examined in Singapore [13].

8.12.2 Adapters to Gather Information from any Human or Machine Source

The role of the interface engine and adapters is to transform all data into XML on a Web information bus. This allows standards-based Web technologies and open source tools to be applied to ongoing PSPAT enhancement.

PSPAT has an interface engine and adapters designed to support a wide variety of interface types:
- XML remote procedure calls used for system integration over IP networks
- HL7 transactions used to transport medical data between medical information systems
- SQL interfaces designed to interact with any SQL database, e.g., XX
- Custom interfaces of any type for specialized systems such as medical devices or robots

The strategic goal of PSPAT is to reduce integration maintenance costs by at least an order of magnitude.

This is critical, as new process improvement targets may require acquisition of data from new systems on an ongoing basis. The software architecture for PSPAT in the UMMC is based on open source software developed on Web services protocols (Fig. 8.5).

8.12.3 MER: Virtual Information Repository for the Workflow Engine Access

A key concept for management of process workflows is that a package of information flows with the patient through every point in the perioperative process. Updating that package shows the real-time state of the patient in process sufficient for the workflow engine to determine what step of the process the patient is in, whether a step in the process is complete, if conditions are met that are necessary to move to the next step, or to ask a specialist to tell the system what the next step should be. This package or MER captures essential real-time data necessary to efficiently and safely manage patient flow.

This package concept is an essential component of the architecture for Boeing Computer Systems and follows an airplane or missile through the entire assembly line process. It is stored in a virtual repository in that primary data resides in hundreds of heterogeneous financial, design, and factory automation systems throughout the Boeing Company. The concept was refined through work with the NIST Automated Manufacturing Research Facility (AMRF) [6] and Titan Systems Corp [35]. It is here extended to health care.

MER information is the fuel for workflow engine processing. The workflow engine will seek out the required information from multiple data sources related to each step the patient goes through in the perioperative process. These sources include, but are not limited to, the electronic medical record used house wide, the perioperative software system, the pharmacy software system, the clinical laboratory software system, the picture archiving system (PACS) used for accessing digitized images, and others. Having user interfaces for the workflow engine Web based, PDA based, and wireless, will provide for easy access to any data source from any location to obtain whatever information is needed for the current step of the workflow process.

8.12.4 A Rules Engine to Provide Intelligent Agent Support for the Workflow Engine

The rules engine maintains a state network or a set of constraints representing medical policies so that at any time (present or historical) the state of all patients

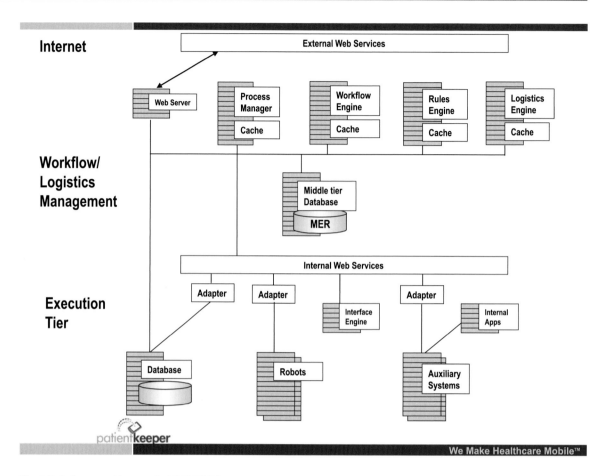

Fig. 8.5 Software architecture for PSPAT [37]

for which data has been received is known. Therefore, upon receipt of new data, the network is updated to reflect any changes in patient, staff, operating room, equipment, or supplies state.

Additionally, actions are defined for rules that have become satisfied. The rules engine is designed to work in conjunction with a physician mobile application platform that will run clinician applications and display appropriate alerts, reminders, and requests for information. The rules incorporated in such applications push them to the level of intelligent agents.

In addition, since the rules engine can store the state network of information for all patients in the perioperative process, it can detect scheduling and other issues across all patients in real time. This is achieved by checking the state of patient data extracted from underlying databases that are accessed through adapters.

Rules may be modified, extended, or included to accommodate new medical insights, hospital, or governmental policies. As a result, the rules environment can evolve with human input to maximize patient throughput, efficiency, and safety of the perioperative process.

8.12.5 An Alerting System to Ensure Timely Completion of Clinical Events

The workflow engine will use as a service a comprehensive alerting system to send messages of any type to any device type, supported by the rules system. It has the additional capability of sending a dynamic query form to an external human interface for data the rules engine needs to process a clinical pathway. In essence, these are "smart alerts." The alerting system can incorporate remote telemedicine experts into the surgery process as required.

8.12.6 A Reporting System to Access Outcomes Data in Real Time

The MER stores the state of each patient in a comprehensive clinical data repository and keeps a record of important state transitions for future analysis. This allows the development of queries to determine improvement in outcomes over time with respect to patient care, efficiency of scheduling and utilization of resources, and the frequency of adverse events detected in the perioperative systems processes.

8.12.7 A Logistics Subsystem to Manage Inventory

The workflow engine orchestrates processes and manages communication of needs and requirements to external systems. It assures that required inventory is on hand to support scheduled surgery and manages reorder of consumable supplies.

8.12.8 Web-Based Telemedicine View

The PSPAT rules engine has the capability of dynamically generating Web-based views of all clinical data, processes, and process states. It can also generate dynamic applications to request or transmit data to any human or machine participant in the perioperative process. This capability will allow external human observers or participants in the perioperative process to view process flow inside the operating room.

8.13 Research Directions

PSPAT will continue to be a proof of concept effort without focused research in the areas of interoperability of medical systems and additional work in the development of open source Web services based protocols appropriate for clinical models like surgery. Work

in this area has been promising; although there is a need for a dedicated surgical extensible markup language that will make brokering information between surgery-based systems and technology relatively easy and inexpensive. This section will discuss the importance of Web services technology to the advancement of technology in surgery.

8.14 Web Services

Some of the current interfaces in health care, particularly financial interfaces, are still batch oriented. The majority of clinical system interfaces are point-to-point, using HL7 version 2–formatted messages. These are difficult to implement and maintain because the HL7 version 2 standard specifies format, but not the semantics of the data put into formatted areas. As a result, every interface in unique and it is sometimes impossible to overcome semantic differences in the meaning of data items as they exist in disparate systems.

HL7 version 3 specifications are based on the HL7 RIM object model and specify structure, semantics, and constraints on data to improve system interoperability. The HL7 standard also specifies XML implementations useful for processing transactions on the Web. The concept of HL7 EHR services that could be used generically for any EHR to access data in any other EHR is in the early stages of analysis and design. It is, however, fundamental to true interoperability of clinical systems and medical devices and would facilitate tight coupling of systems via Web transactions (phase 3 in Fig. 8.6).

Full specification of HL7 version 3 Web services would streamline implementations of PSPAT by allowing the PSPAT workflow engine to more easily orchestrate behaviors across disparate health care systems

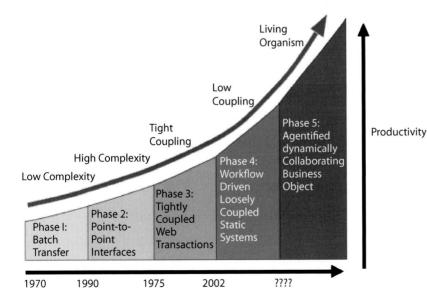

Fig. 8.6 Improved enterprise integration leads to enhanced interoperability, more access to critical functionality, lower implementation and maintenance costs, plug and play architectures, and more flexible and intelligent systems [21, 33]

and medical devices. Early work is underway jointly by HL7 and the Object Management Group [27], and a software factory implementation using the latest Visual Studio tooling has been specified by Microsoft [2].

The highest stage of interoperability (phase 5 in Fig. 8.6) would allow agents to implement goal-seeking behavior based on collaborative orchestration of higher-level services provided by one or more workflow engines [21]. These will be essential to future military systems now being prototyped using autonomous robots as surgeons [12].

8.15   Conclusion

Work on the Operating Room of the Future at the University of Maryland Medical System in partnership with technical experts from PatientKeeper and the University of Tilburg, using approaches described above is the first known prototype implementation of a standards based workflow engine in an operating room suite to monitor, manage, and improve throughput, while enhancing patient safety and patient care.

Extensive implementation of heavyweight, proprietary systems in health care has created islands of automation that create excessive expense, high cost of technology change, crippled functionality due to lack of integration of disparate systems, extremely high rates of medical error, and low quality of patient care and patient satisfaction. It is possible to use low-cost, open source, standards-based approaches in the implementation of operating facilities information systems infrastructure. High levels of integration using a Web services bus and proven components can enhance functionality, reliability, performance, and patient safety.

The advent of new technologies including RFID, mobile/wireless technologies, automated business process management (internet workflow systems and intelligent agents), SOAs, and business process management (BPM) opens up new ways of automating business processes, overcoming barriers to technology adoption, and resolving problematic issues like patient, staff, and equipment location [25]. Total situational awareness of events, timing, and location of critical health care activities makes possible real time process improvement by (1) anticipating future behaviors of complex systems, (2) displaying the probable futures of complex operations to all affected personnel, (3) generating self-organizing change in behaviors of humans and machines, (4) erasing a possible negative future outcome, and (5) replacing it with a modified future outcome that meets organizational goals.

The RECIPE approach makes it possible to unobtrusively introduce real time process improvement into an operational health care environment through:

- RFID tracking of patients, staff, supplies, instruments, equipment—accumulating baseline data
- Analysis of patient flow bottlenecks and development of process improvements targets
- Manual testing of process improvements
- Integration of a standards-based workflow management system into the enterprise information technology infrastructure
- Small incremental process improvements introduced through the workflow engine with rapid fine-tuning
- Make disruption visible proactively
- Orchestrate human and machine behavior to anticipate and resolve problems
- Dynamic application generation: real-time support for workflow engine to obtain information needed at any step of process

The potential gains from this approach are enormous in terms of improved efficiency and patient safety. Simply understanding the process of workflow enhancement of clinical processes generated a 100% improvement in supply and instrument readiness in a large operating room suite. Full implementation of an automated workflow facility with integration into production clinical systems could induce a radical reinvention of clinical process integration, resulting in improved patient outcomes, an enhanced staff working environment, significant cost reduction, and enhancement of institutional revenue.

Even more important, effective implementation of the RECIPE approach would automate feedback mechanisms for routine, systematic, ongoing enhancement of clinical processes. Implementation of intelligent automated systems in other domains with computerized feedback loops have led to emergent architectures with higher adaptability, capability, extensibility, and maintainability than could be initially conceived by the original designers of such systems [9, 11]. By doing so, RECIPE open ups ways to move away from medical production systems, and facilitate ad hoc, autonomic workflows that are capable of adjusting themselves to new situations, monitor and recover from disruptions, and deal with attacks from anywhere.

References

1. Allen S (2004) Emergency room recovery. Boston Globe, Boston, p A1
2. Anonymous (2005) A software factory approach to HL7 version 3 solutions. Microsoft with Blueprint Technologies, Redmond, Wash.
3. Anyanwu K et al (2003) Health care enterprise process development and integration. J Res Pract Inf Technol 35:83–98

4. Arthur WB (1994) On the evolution of complexity, in complexity: metaphors, models, and reality. In: Cowan GA, Pines D, Meltzer D (eds) Proceedings volume XIX, Sante Fe Institute studies in the science of complexity. Addison-Wesley, Boston

5. Balas EA et al (2000) Improving preventive care by prompting physicians. Arch Intern Med 160:301–308

6. Barkmeyer E, Lo J (1989) Experience with IMDAS in the automated manufacturing research facility. National Institute of Standards and Technology, Gaithersburg, Md.

7. Beyea SC, Kilbridge P (2003) Setting a research agenda on patient safety in surgical settings. Semin Laparosc Surg 10:79–83

8. Brooks RA (1991) How to build complete creatures rather than isolated cognitive simulators. In: VanLehn K (ed) Architectures for intelligence. Lawrence Erlbaum, Hillsdale, N.J., pp 225–239

9. Brooks RA (1991) Intelligence without representation. Artif Intell 47:139–159

10. Dadam P, Reichert M, Kuhn K (2000) Clinical workflows – the killer application for process-oriented information systems. In: BIS 2000 – proceedings of the 4th International Conference on Business Information Systems, Poznan, Poland. Springer, Berlin Heidelberg New York

11. Defense Advanced Research Projects Agency (2004) One Year Countdown to Grand Challenge 2005. DARPA Publishes Rules, Team Application Status Report. Defense Advanced Research Projects Agency, Arlington, Va.

12. Defense Advanced Research Projects Agency (2003) DARPA, Operating Room of the Future Workshop, Executive Summary. Defense Advanced Research Projects Agency, Arlington, Va., pp 1–2

13. Dhaliwal JS et al (1997) Using enterprise modeling to reengineer health care processes. SIGGROUP Bull 18:51–53

14. Exavera Technologies (2004) Exavera, eShepard FAQ (frequently asked questions). Exavera Technologies, Portsmouth, N.H.

15. Gatersleben MR, van der Weij SW (1999) Analysis and simulation of passenger flows in an airport terminal. In: Proceedings of the 31st Conference on Winter Simulation: Simulation—a bridge to the future. ACM, Phoenix

16. Goldratt EM, Cox J (1994) The goal: a process of ongoing improvement, 2nd rev. edn. North River, Great Barrington, Mass

17. Henckels C (2003) Wrong-site surgery: a study of medical misadventure claims. New Zealand Accident Compensation Corporation Medical Misadventure Unit, Wellington

18. Hinchley A (2003) Understanding version 3: a primer on the HL7 version 3 communication standard. Understanding HL7 Series. Mönch, Munich

19. Institute of Medicine (US) Committee on Quality of Health Care in America (2004) Patient safety: achieving a new standard for care. National Academies Press, Washington, D.C.

20. Larsen RA et al (1989) Improved perioperative antibiotic use and reduced surgical wound infections through use of computer decision analysis. Infect Control Hosp Epidemiol 10:316–320

21. Maamar Z, Sutherland J (2000) Toward intelligent business objects: focusing on techniques to enhance BPs that exhibit goal-oriented behaviors. Comm ACM 40:99–101

22. Manolescu DA, Paul S (2003) An evaluation framework for workflow engines. Personal communication

23. Marsland S, Buchan I (2004) Clinical quality needs complex adaptive systems and machine learning. In: Fieschi M (ed) MEDINFO 2004. IOS, Amsterdam

24. McGlynn EA et al (2003) The quality of health care delivered to adults in the United States. N Engl J Med 348:2635–2645

25. Minear MN, Sutherland J (2003) Medical informatics—a catalyst for operating room transformation. Semin Laparosc Surg 10:71–78

26. Ogunnaike BA, Ray WH (1994) Process dynamics, modeling, and control. Topics in chemical engineering. Oxford University Press, Oxford

27. Object Management Group and Health Level Seven (2005) Object Management Group begin joint health care software services standardization work: combined effort leverages strengths of each organization. OMG Press Release 8 March 2005, Needham, Mass.

28. Paul S, Park E, Chaar J (1998) Essential requirements for a workflow standard. In: Patel D, Sutherland J, Miller J (eds) Business object design and implementation II: OOPSLA '96, OOPSLA '97, and OOPSLA '98 Proceedings. Springer, Berlin Heidelberg New York, pp 100–108

29. Paul S, Park E, Chaar J (1997) RainMan: a workflow system for the Internet. IBM T.J. Watson Research Center, Yorktown Heights, N.Y.

30. Sandberg WS, Ganous TJ, Steiner C (2003) Setting a research agenda for perioperative systems design. Semin Laparosc Surg 10:57–70

31. Starfield B (2000) Is US health really the best in the world? JAMA 2000. 284:483–485

32. Sutherland J, Alpert S (1999) Big Workflow for enterprise applications. In: Patel D, Sutherland J, Miller J (eds) Business object design and implementation III: OOPSLA '99 workshop proceedings. Springer, Berlin Heidelberg New York

33. Sutherland J, van den Heuvel WJ (2002) Enterprise application integration and complex adaptive systems: could system integration and cooperation be improved with agentified enterprise components? Comm ACM 45:59–64

34. Sutherland J et al (2005) RECIPE for REal-time proCess ImProvement in health care: putting the health care enterprise on autopilot, in future of health technology. In: Bushko R (ed) Future of Health Technology. Cambridge, Cambridge, Mass.

35. Sutherland JV (1989) Architectural vision for manufacturing and 3CI support. Object Databases, Cambridge, Mass.

36. Sutherland JV (2004) RECIPE for REal time proCess ImProvement in health care. In: Proceedings of the Future of Health Technology Summit. Massachusetts Institute of Technology, Cambridge

37. Sutherland JV (2004) RECIPE for REal time proCess ImProvement in health care. In: 13th Annual Physician–Computer Connection Symposium. American Society for Medical Directors of Information Systems (AMDIS). Rancho Bernardo, Calif.

38. Thompson TG, Brailer DJ (2004) The decade of health information technology: delivering consumer-centric and information-rich health care – framework for strategic action. US Departmetn of Health and Human Services, Washington, D.C.

39. Zimmerman B, Plsek P, Lindberg C (1998) Edgeware: insights from complexity science for health care leader. VHA, Irvine, Tex.

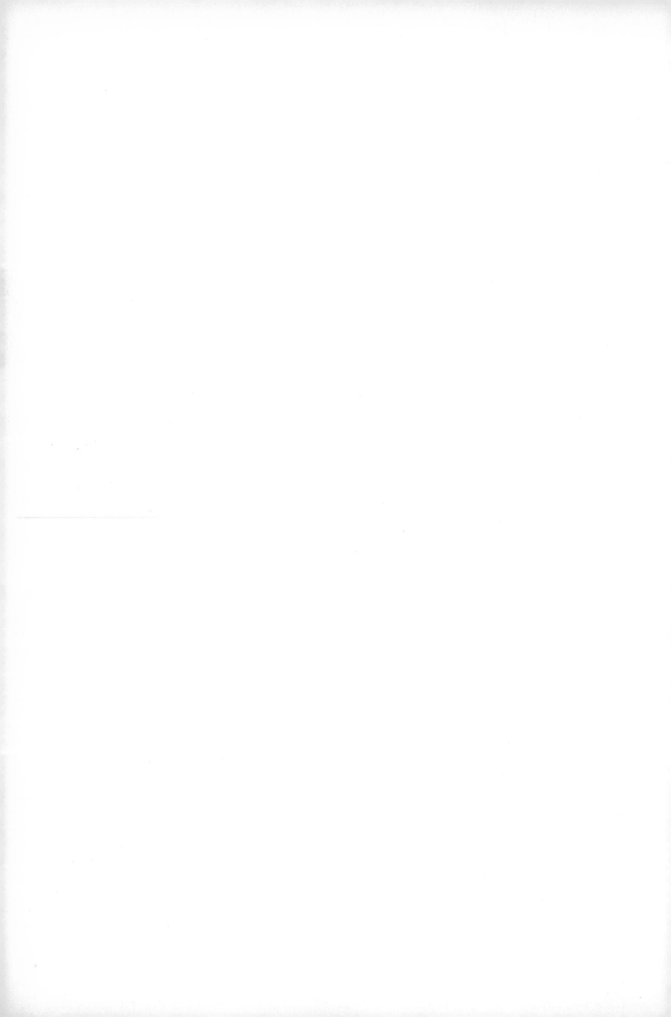

Part III
Robotics and Novel Surgical Approaches

Robotics in General Surgery: Today and Tomorrow

Federico Moser and Santiago Horgan

9.1 Introduction

The world of surgery, having so long been isolated from computers, is evolving. The adoption of robotic technology is widespread. It covers the spectrum of surgical specialties and crosses international boundaries. More than 10,000 operations have been performed using the da Vinci® surgical system. General surgeons, urologists, neurosurgeons, thoracic surgeons, cardiovascular surgeons, gynecologists, and vascular surgeons alike are using the system. The range of robotic cases ranges from the simplest cholecystectomy to the most complex mitral valve repair. An informal survey conducted in 2004 by our university showed that approximately 200 systems in the United States, 60 systems in Europe, and 6 systems in Asia are currently in clinical use. At the University of Illinois at Chicago, we have performed more than 300 robotic-assisted procedures (Table 9.1). In this chapter, we review the current application of robotics in general surgery.

Table 9.1 Robotic-assisted procedures performed at the University of Illinois

Procedure	Number of cases
Cholecystectomy	1
Roux en-Y gastric bypass	110
Adjustable gastric banding	30
Heller myotomy	50
Nissen fundoplication	5
Epiphrenic diverticulectomy	6
Total esophagectomy	18
Esophageal leiomyoma resection	3
Pyloroplasty	1
Gastroyeyunostomy	2
Transduodenal sphincteroplasty	2
Adrenalectomy	10
Donor nephrectomy	120

9.2 Cholecystectomy

Since the first robotic-assisted cholecystectomy was performed in 1997 by Himpens et al. in Belgium [1], several case series were reported in the literature [2, 3]. The authors of these studies did not find any significant advantages over conventional laparoscopic surgery when using the robotic system to perform the operation. They stated that the need for a specially trained operating room staff was an unnecessary hindrance for a low-complexity procedure. They also stated that the operating room costs were higher with the robotic system, due to more expensive instrumentation, robot time, and longer case time. In addition, they indicated that it was extremely difficult to perform a cholangiogram with the system in place due to the large footprint and bulk of the robotic arms. At this time, there are no case studies or randomized controlled trials large enough to suggest the expected decrease in complications of cholecystectomy, such as common bile duct (CBD) injury. In conclusion, we postulate that the advantages of robotic technology may have potential use in advanced procedures such as repair of the common bile duct after injury, but that current evidence does not support the routine application of this technology in laparoscopic cholecystectomy.

9.3 Bariatric Surgery

The field of bariatric surgery benefited greatly from the introduction of minimally invasive techniques. Robotic-assisted surgery represents a small but growing subset of minimally invasive surgical applications that enables surgeons to perform bariatric procedures with minimal alteration of their current laparoscopic or open technique. A survey of surgeons in 2003 showed that only 11 surgeons in the United States were currently using a robotic surgical system for bariatric surgery [4]. The reason for this is the small number of bariatric cases performed laparoscopically (10%) in the United States and the limited number of institutions with a robotic system. The first robotic-assisted adjustable gastric banding was reported in 1999 [5], and the first-ever robotically assisted gastric bypass in September 2000 by our group [6].

9.3.1 Robotic-Assisted Roux-en-Y Gastric Bypass

The procedure that benefits most from robotic assistance in the field of bariatric surgery is the gastric bypass. Our group currently uses the system to perform a robotic-assisted, hand-sewn gastrojejunostomy for completion of the laparoscopic Roux-en-Y gastric bypass procedure. The operative room is set up as shown in (Fig. 9.1). The first part of the opera-

tion is performed laparoscopically; a small pouch and a 120-cm limb are created. After this, the robot is put in place and a running two-layer, hand-sewn antecolic antegastric gastrojejunal anastomosis is performed. We believe that performing a hand-sewn anastomosis offers the best method to decrease the risk of leak. We recently completed analyzing the data of our robotic bariatric surgeon and a surgeon at an outside institution. Both surgeons were junior faculty and were well within the steep learning curve of the minimally invasive approach. They have now completed close to 200 procedures without an anastomotic leak. They have also experienced significantly fewer strictures than the 9–14% expected rate of circular stapler anastomotic techniques [7, 8]. Performing a hand-sewn anastomosis also eliminates the requirement of passing a stapler anvil down the esophagus (avoiding the risk of esopha-

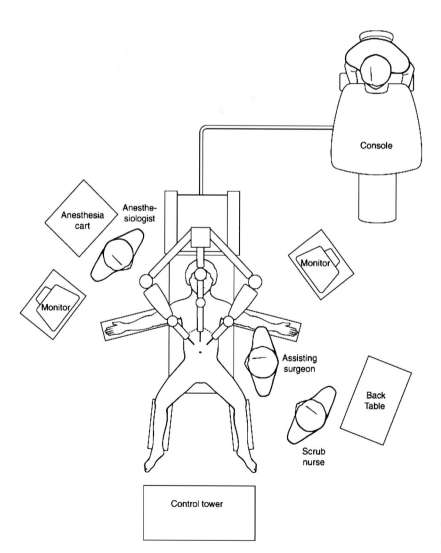

Fig. 9.1 Operating room set up for esophageal surgery and gastric bypass

geal injury) or adding an additional stapler line after passing the anvil transgastric. In addition, our survey of national robotic surgeons revealed that 107 cases of robotic-assisted Roux-en-Y gastric bypasses were performed by seven surgeons in the United States in 2003 [4]. The main utility of the robotic system was found to be in creating the gastrojejunostomy, the articulating wrists, three-dimensional view, and motion scaling, allow a precise hand-sewn anastomosis [4] (Fig. 9.2). This was most notable in patients with a high basal metabolic rate ([BMI] greater than 60 or super obese) and/or those patients with an enlarged left hepatic lobe, which greatly decreases the working area beneath the liver. Regarding operative time, surgeons having an experience greater than 20 cases reported that preparation for the robot can be decreased to as little as 6 min and robotic work time can also diminish by 50% [4].

Our institutional experience and that of the surgeons who responded to our survey is that robotically assisted hand-sewn gastrojejunostomy is superior to any currently available minimally invasive anastomotic technique. This technique has the potential to diminish the leak, stricture, and mortality rates of this procedure [4]. However, larger studies conducted in prospective randomized fashion still need to be performed to verify our currently perceived clinical advantages.

9.3.2 Robotic-Assisted Adjustable Gastric Banding

Robotic-assisted adjustable gastric banding is also performed at select institutions. Three of 11 surveyed robotic-assisted bariatric surgeons in the United States were using the da Vinci® System in 2003 [4]. At the University of Illinois at Chicago, we began randomizing patients to robotic or laparoscopic adjustable gastric banding placement in 2001. We found similar outcomes in length of hospital stay and weight loss, although the operative time was significantly longer in the robotic group [4]. In our experience, we were able to distinguish the advantages of the robotic approach from the disadvantage of increased operative time. It was apparent that patients with BMI greater than 60 would benefit most. In these patients, the increased torque on conventional laparoscopic instruments makes precise operative technique vastly more difficult. Robotic instruments are thicker (8 mm), and the mechanical system is able to deliver more force while operating in these patients with thick abdominal walls. The mechanical power provided by the robotic system provides relief to the operating surgeon, eliminating the struggle to maintain instrument position or counter the torque from rotating instruments around the fixed pivot point. In addition, the increased intra-abdominal fat content and size of the viscera, especially the liver, in these patients leaves a much smaller operative field. In this situation, the robotic manipulation of the articulating instruments in small working areas provides significant advantage. Given these observations, we are currently using the robotic system in patients with a BMI greater than 60.

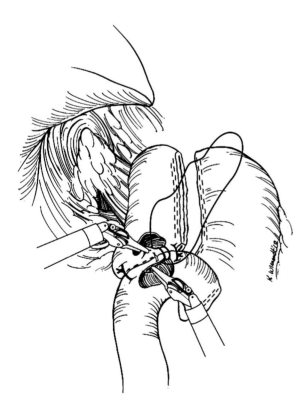

Fig. 9.2 Gastrojejunal anastomosis for gastric bypass

9.3.3 Robotic-Assisted Biliary Pancreatic Diversion with Duodenal Switch

The third bariatric procedure being perfomed is robotic-assisted biliary pancreatic diversion with duodenal switch (BPD-DS). Three surgeons are currently using the robot for this procedure, Drs. Ranjan and Debra Sudan from Creighton Hospital in Omaha, and Dr. Gagner from Mount Sinai in New York [4]. Most reports describe performing the duodenojejunal anastomosis with robotic-assistance. No comparative data have been reported. However, the stated advantages are the system's ability to complete an otherwise difficult and advanced laparoscopic maneuver with greater ease and more precision, with no untoward effects.

9.4   Esophageal Surgery

Advanced esophageal procedures, previously requiring large open and at times thoracic incisions, can now be performed minimally invasively providing decreased pain and hospital time to the patient. The general rules for all the esophageal procedures performed via the abdomen are similar. For the trocar placement, the first port placed is 12 mm, and is placed using a gasless optical technique. It is positioned two fingerbreadths lateral to the umbilicus and one palm width inferior to the left subcostal margin. The position of this port is optimal for viewing the gastroesophageal junction, and the size is appropriate for the robotic camera. One 8-mm robotic port is then placed just inferior to the left costal margin in the midclavicular line. A 12-mm port is then inserted again inferior to the left costal margin but in the anterior axillary line. The large size of this port is essential for the insertion of stapling devices, and clip appliers by the assistant if needed. The extreme lateral position is necessary for proper retraction, and avoidance of collisions with the robotic arms. A Nathanson liver retractor is then inserted just inferior to the xiphoid process. The liver is then retracted anteriorly, exposing the esophageal hiatus, and another 8-mm robotic port is inserted inferior to the right costal margin in the midclavicular line. The room setting and the position of the robotic system is similar in all the advanced esophageal procedures (Fig. 9.1). In the following esophageal procedures, with exception of the Nissen fundoplication, we found benefits in the robotic assisted approach when comparing with the laparoscopic technique. Although the Nissen fundoplication is a very useful procedure to learn robotic surgery, in our experience it has been shown to prolong the operative time with similar postoperative results.

9.4.1   Heller Myotomy

Achalasia, a disease of unknown etiology, results in failure of lower esophageal sphincter (LES) relaxation and aperistalsis. The incidence is about 1 in 100,000 in North America. Options for medical management include medication, botulinum toxin injection, and balloon dilatation. None of nonsurgical treatments have been as successful as surgical myotomy. Many years after Heller performed the first surgical myotomy, the minimally invasive surgical techniques became the gold standard of the surgical treatment for the achala-

sia. However, the surgeons are still hampered by their inability to have flexible instruments and high-definition video imaging. The robotic system is ideally suited for advanced esophageal surgery, and we have applied this technology in our surgical approach to achalasia. The myotomy is extended a minimum of 6 cm proximally and 1–2 cm distally onto the gastric fundus. Failure to achieve adequate proximal dissection of the esophagus with a subsequent short myotomy is the most common reason for failure. Therefore, the dissection of the esophagus should extend well into the thorax in order to complete the myotomy. The laparoscopic approach in this small area is often difficult and frequently the visual field is obscured by the instrumentation. The articulating wrists of the robot enable the surgeon to operate in the narrow field around the thoracic esophagus without this limitation. Perforation of the esophageal mucosa, seen in 5–10% of laparoscopic cases independent of the surgeon's experience, is the most feared complication when performing a Heller myotomy. The three-dimensional view with ×12 magnification and the natural tremor of the surgeon's hand eliminated through electronic filtering of the robotic system allow each individual muscular fiber to be visualized and divided ensuring a proper myotomy, diminishing dramatically the incidence of perforation (Fig. 9.3). Following the myotomy and crural closure, we complete a Dor fundoplication. In the last 4 years, our group performed 50 robotically assisted myotomy for achalasia at our institution. In our series, we have not experienced a single perforation, even though many of our patients were treated with Botox preoperatively; a similar number of cases have been compiled by Dr. Melvin at Ohio State University, with similar results. The average length of hospital stay is 1.5 days (range: 0.8–4), with no conversions and a 100% success rate. We strongly believe that the robotic-assisted approach will be the gold standard for Heller myotomy in the near future.

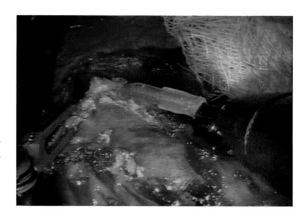

Fig. 9.3 Robotic myotomy of circular esophageal fibers

9.4.2 Resection of Epiphrenic Diverticulum

Epiphrenic diverticulum is an uncommon entity that most frequently occurs on the right side of the distal 10 cm of the esophagus. The pathogenesis of esophageal diverticula remains controversial [9]. The most common symptoms are dysphagia, heartburn, and regurgitation of undigested food particles. Surgery is indicated in symptomatic patients, and a myotomy at the time of the excision is recommended when abnormal motility is present. Longer instruments and reticulating wrists allow surgeons to extend the dissection deep into the thorax for more proximal diverticula and to operate in tight quarters, manipulating the esophagus without causing undue tension or torque on this structure. The robotic system clearly facilitates the dissection of the neck of the diverticulum when compared with conventional laparoscopic instruments. Once the diverticulum neck is identified and dissected free, the diverticulum is resected using an endoscopic linear stapler. Endoscopy is used to aid in identification of the diverticulum intraoperatively, and for inspection of the staple line following removal. When preoperative testing reveals a motility disorder, a myotomy with a Dor fundoplication is performed. The robotic-assisted approach via the abdomen has been used in six patients within our institution. As with myotomy for achalasia, we feel the robotic system markedly improves the accuracy which this can be performed thereby reducing the chance of mucosal perforation.

9.4.3 Total Esophagectomy

The benefits of using laparoscopic technique for total esophagectomy have been already reported [10, 11]. The laparoscopic transhiatal dissection of the esophageal body near the pulmonary vein, the aorta, and the parietal pleura is very challenging. Our first robotic-assisted transhiatal esophagectomy was reported in 2003 [12]. For this procedure, the thoracic portion of the operations (via the abdomen) is undertaken with the robotic system, and one assistant port. The cervical anastomosis is carried out with an open cervical incision in all cases. The articulated instruments using the robotic system allow precise blunt and sharp dissection of the intrathoracic esophageal attachments. The benefits of robotics are maximized in this surgery in that the reticulating writs allow the surgeon to navigate such a narrow space of dissection. Because of this reticulation, the shaft of the instruments is out of the surgeon's view, keeping the field clear. The three-dimensional image and the chance of magnification of the operative field view provide extreme detail and clarity. When scarring is present, making tissue less yielding to blunt dissec-

tion, the articulating hook makes possible a safe periesophageal dissection, preventing bleeding and trauma. Additionally, the robotics instruments are 7.5 cm longer than are standard laparoscopic instruments; therefore, it is possible a greater proximal mobilization beyond the level of the carina and a thoracoscopic approach is not necessary. With the esophagus fully mobilized, the stomach is then tubularized along the lesser curve, using several fires of a Linear Cutting Stapler (Ethicon, Cincinnati, Ohio). The esophagus is removed through the neck, and the anastomosis is performed. A total of 14 patients have undergone robotically assisted total esophagectomy for a diagnosis of high-grade dysplasia at our institution. In our series, the total operative time was 279 (175–360) min, including robotic setup time. Our last five cases averaged 210 min (range 175–210). The intraoperative average blood loss for the combined robotic and open cervical portions of the operations was 43 (10–60) ml. There were no intraoperative complications, and no patients developed laryngeal nerve injury postoperatively. The hospital stay averaged 8 (6–8) days. There have been no deaths, and our current average follow up is 264 (45–531) days. We believe that with minimal blood loss, short hospital and ICU stays, and lack of mortality, robotically assisted transhiatal esophagectomy has proven to a safe and effective operation. However, randomized controlled trials need to be conducted to inspect oncologic integrity if this operation is to be performed in patients with diagnoses other than high-grade dysplasia.

9.4.4 Esophageal Leiomyoma

Leiomyoma is the most common benign mesenchymal esophageal tumor, representing up to 80% of benign esophageal tumors. Anatomically these neoplasms are localized to the middle and lower thirds of the esophagus, in most cases as a single lesion [13]. The most common symptoms include dysphagia and atypical chest pain. Surgical intervention is indicated not only for pain but also in asymptomatic patients in order to prevent the excessive growth that can complicate patient well-being and future surgical resection. For resection of a leiomyoma, the patient is placed in the left lateral decubitus position and a robotic-assisted thoracoscopy is performed via five trocars. Circumferential dissection of the esophagus is performed using the hook electrocautery robotic extension. The articulated instruments allow the surgeon to place the grasper behind the esophagus without producing torque, which is frequent with rigid thoracoscopic instruments and facilitate a safe dissection of tumors that lie near the azygous vein. The isolation of the tumor starts by transecting the longitudinal muscular layer (myotomy), us-

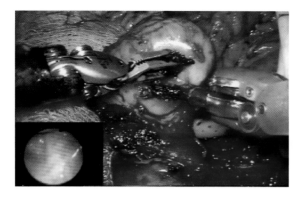

Fig. 9.4 Robotic-assisted enucleation of a leiomyoma

ing the articulating robotic electrocautery. Then, blunt and sharp dissection is used to enucleate the tumor from the esophageal wall (Fig. 9.4). The articulating wrists allow a precise closure of the myotomy in a running fashion to complete the procedure. In our series, we have not seen mucosal injury, which we attribute to the better visualization, precise dissection afforded by the articulated instruments, and tremor control provided by the robotic system [14].

9.5   Pancreatic Surgery

The application of minimally invasive techniques for pancreatic surgery remains in its infancy. Since the first endocrine pancreatic tumor resection was reported by Gagner and Sussman in 1996 [15, 16], only one robotic-assisted pancreatic tumor resection case was reported by Melvin in 2003 [17]. Melvin's group has also reported the experience of pancreatic duct reconstruction after open pancreaticoduodenectomy. Although there are no reported data available, Giulianotti et al. from Italy have performed more than 20 robotic Whipple resections with very good results. Robotic pancreatic resection is feasible, but further advances in techniques and technology are necessary and future experience will determine the real benefits of this approach.

9.6   Gastric Surgery

A limited number of robotic-assisted gastric surgeries were reported in the United States. These include pyloroplasties, gastric mass resections, and gastrojejunostomies [6, 18]. In Japan, a country with high incidence of gastric cancer, the laparoscopic treatment for early gastric cancer has been used with good results [19]. Hashizume et al. reported the use of the robotic system

to perform surgery for gastric cancer. The benefits of the EndoWrist, the scaling and the tremor filtering, was found to be extremely useful when performing wedge resections, intragastric resections, and distal gastrectomies [20]. Even though the initial results can be encouraging, more experience is required to establish the role of the robotic system in the gastric surgery.

9.7   Colorectal Surgery

The introduction of laparoscopy to colorectal surgery extended benefits of minimally invasive techniques to this arena. These benefits include shorter hospital stay, earlier return to activities, etc. A robotic-assisted approach in the field of colorectal surgery is very promising, even though the current experience is very limited. There are reports on right hemicolectomy, sigmoid colectomy, rectopexy, anterior resection, and abdominoperineal resection [21–23]. Surgeons agree that the robot can be very useful in rectal surgery. Fazio et al., from the Cleveland Clinic, compared robotic with laparoscopic approaches for colectomy in a small group of patients; they concluded that robotic colectomy is feasible and safe, but operative time is increased [24]. In conclusion, robotic assistance, as in others fields of surgery, may facilitate complex colorectal surgeries, but more experience is still necessary.

9.8   Adrenalectomy

The first laparoscopic endocrine surgery experiences published in the literature were the laparoscopic adrenalectomies performed by Gagner in 1992 [25]. Currently, the minimally invasive approach is the recommended standard for the treatment of benign adrenal lesions. In Italy in 1999, Piazza and colleagues published the first robotic-assisted adrenalectomy using the Zeus Aesop [26]. One year later, in August 2000, V. B. Kim and colleagues used the da Vinci® Robotic Surgical System to fully assist an adrenalectomy [2]. Our first robotic-assisted bilateral adrenalectomy was published in 2001 [6]. Brunaud and others prospectively compared standard laparoscopic adrenalectomy and robotic-assisted adrenalectomy in a group of 28 patients. They found the robotic approach seemed to be longer (111 vs. 83 min, $p = 0.057$), but this tendency decreased with surgeon experience. The morbidity and the hospital stay were similar for both groups. In addition, duration of standard laparoscopic adrenalectomy was positively correlated to patient's BMI. This correlation was absent in patients operated on with the da Vinci® system [27]. Objective benefits of robotic vs.

laparoscopic approach have not been demonstrated yet, but even given the limited experience available, the robotic system seems to be very useful for adrenalectomy in overweight and obese patients.

9.9   Donor Nephrectomy

Living kidney donation represents an important source for patients with end-stage renal disease (ESRD), and has emerged as an appealing alternative to cadaveric donation. Furthermore, within the last decade, laparoscopic donor nephrectomy has replaced the conventional open approach, and has gained surgeon and patients acceptance.

The first laparoscopic living donor nephrectomy was attempted to alleviate the shortage of kidneys for transplantation and to reduce the hospitalization and recuperation time associated to with open nephrectomy [28]. The outcomes reported for the laparoscopic technique were similar to the open operation, adding all the advantages of minimally invasive procedures [29]. The reduction of postoperative pain, shorter hospital stay, better cosmetic results, and shorter convalescence time are increasing the acceptance of the donors with the subsequent expansion of donor pool [30, 31].

We started performing the robotic hand–assisted living donor nephrectomy utilizing the da Vinci® Surgical System (Intuitive Surgical, Sunny Valley, Calif.) in January 2001. Our technique is hand-assisted using the

LAP DISC (Ethicon, Cincinnati, Ohio) (Fig. 9.5). The utilization of a hand-assisted device like the LAP DISC allows for faster removal of the kidney to decrease warm ischemia time [32]. Another advantage of having the hand inside the abdomen is rapid control in case of bleeding, and avoidance of excessive manipulation of the kidney, which is otherwise required in the removal of the kidney with an extraction bag. The robotic system provides the benefits of a minimally invasive approach without giving up the dexterity, precision and intuitive movements of open surgery.

A helical CT angiogram with three-dimensional reconstruction of the kidney is performed on all patients to evaluate abnormalities in the parenchyma, the collecting system, and renal vascular anatomy. The reconstruction is a useful roadmap to identify the presence of multiple renal arteries. The room setup is critical in our current operation (Fig. 9.6). Two assisting surgeons are required; one surgeon has his or her right hand inside the patient, and the second surgeon exchanges the robotic instruments and assists the operative surgeon through the 12-mm trocar.

Since the beginning of our experience, we have implemented the policy of routinely harvesting the left kidney, regardless of the presence of vascular anomalies, to take advantage of the longer length of the left renal vein. The presence of multiple renal arteries or veins has not been a problem for robotic-assisted approach. We performed a study with 112 patients who underwent robotic-assisted LLDN, where the patient population was divided into two groups based on the

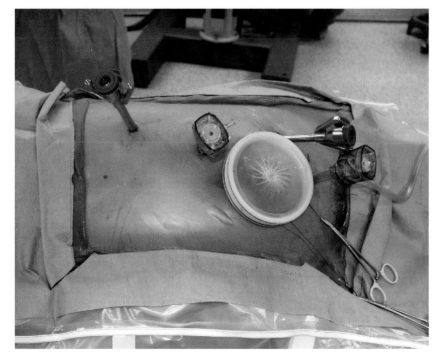

Fig. 9.5 Trocar and hand-port placement for donor nephrectomy

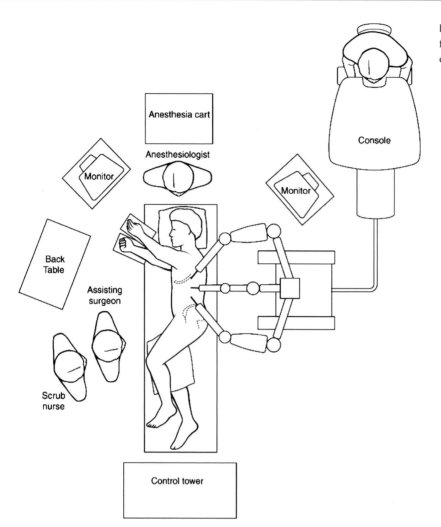

Fig. 9.6 Operating room set up for nephrectomy and adrenalectomy

presence of normal renal vascular anatomy (group A: $n = 81$, 72.3%) or multiple renal arteries or veins (group B: $n = 31$, 27.7%). No significant difference in mortality, morbidity, conversion rate, operative time, blood loss, warm ischemia time, or length of hospital stay was noted between the two groups. The outcome of kidney transplantation in the recipients was also similar in the two groups.

Since we started in 2000, we have improved on our operative technique. We have noticed a statically significant decrease in the operative time ($p < 0.0001$), suggesting experience and confidence of the surgical transplant team. The average operative time dropped from an initial 206 min (range: 120–320 min) in the first 50 cases to 156 min (range: 85–240 min) in the last 50 cases ($p < 0.0001$). The mean warm ischemia time was 87 s (range: 60–120 s). The average estimated blood loss was 50 ml (range: 10–1,500 ml). The length of hospital stay averaged 2 days (range: 1–8 days). One-

year patient and graft survivals were 100 and 98%, respectively. In conclusion, our data demonstrates that robotic hand–assisted donor nephrectomy is a safe and effective procedure.

9.10 Conclusion

The introduction of the robotic system in the field of minimally invasive surgery has produced an authentic revolution. Robotic surgery remains still in its infancy, and the limits of its expansion are unpredictable. Nevertheless, the robotic approach has already proved to be safe and feasible in the most complex procedures in general surgery. Currently, clear advantages of robotic technology are proven in surgical procedures where very precise movements in small areas and a good vision of the surgical field are required such as esophageal surgery, bariatric surgery, donor nephrectomies, rectal surgery, etc. However, in the era of evidence-based medicine, larger studies conducted in prospective randomized fashion still need to be performed to verify the perceived clinical benefits. The velocity of the expansion of the robotic-assisted surgery is going to depend on the greater experience of the surgeons and the introduction of more technological advances.

References

1. Jacob BP, Gagner M (2003) Robotics and general surgery. Surg Clin North Am 83:1405–1419

2. Kim VB et al (2002) Early experience with telemanipulative robot-assisted laparoscopic cholecystectomy using da Vinci. Surg Laparosc Endosc Percutan Tech 12:33–40

3. Marescaux J et al (2001) Telerobotic laparoscopic cholecystectomy: initial clinical experience with 25 patients. Ann Surg 234:1–7

4. Jacobsen G, Berger R, Horgan S (2003) The role of robotic surgery in morbid obesity. J Laparoendosc Adv Surg Tech A 13:279–283

5. Cadiere GB et al (1999) The world's first obesity surgery performed by a surgeon at a distance. Obes Surg 9:206–209

6. Horgan S, Vanuno D (2001) Robots in laparoscopic surgery. J Laparoendosc Adv Surg Tech A 11:415–419

7. Papasavas PK et al (2003) Laparoscopic management of complications following laparoscopic Roux-en-Y gastric bypass for morbid obesity. Surg Endosc 17:610–614

8. Perugini RA et al (2003) Predictors of complication and suboptimal weight loss after laparoscopic Roux-en-Y gastric bypass: a series of 188 patients. Arch Surg 138:541–545; discussion 545–546

9. Matthews BD et al (2003) Minimally invasive management of epiphrenic esophageal diverticula. Am Surg 69:465–470; discussion 470

10. Sadanaga N et al (1994) Laparoscopy-assisted surgery: a new technique for transhiatal esophageal dissection. Am J Surg 168:355–357

11. Swanstrom LL, Hansen P (1997) Laparoscopic total esophagectomy. Arch Surg 132:943–947; discussion 947–949

12. Horgan S et al (2003) Robotic-assisted minimally invasive transhiatal esophagectomy. Am Surg 69:624–626

13. Nguyen NT, Alcocer JJ, Luketich JD (2000) Thoracoscopic enucleation of an esophageal leiomyoma. J Clin Gastroenterol 31:89–90

14. Elli E et al (2004) Robotic-assisted thoracoscopic resection of esophageal leiomyoma. Surg Endosc 18:713–716

15. Gagner M, Pomp A, Herrera MF (1996) Early experience with laparoscopic resections of islet cell tumors. Surgery 120:1051–1054

16. Sussman LA, Christie R, Whittle DE (1996) Laparoscopic excision of distal pancreas including insulinoma. Aust NZ J Surg 66:414–416

17. Melvin WS et al (2003) Robotic resection of pancreatic neuroendocrine tumor. J Laparoendosc Adv Surg Tech A 13:33–36

18. Talamini MA et al (2003) A prospective analysis of 211 robotic-assisted surgical procedures. Surg Endosc 17:1521–1524

19. Ohgami M et al (1999) Curative laparoscopic surgery for early gastric cancer: five years experience. World J Surg 23:187–192; discussion 192–193

20. Hashizume M, Sugimachi K (2003) Robot-assisted gastric surgery. Surg Clin North Am 83:1429–1444

21. Rockall TA, Darzi A (2003) Robot-assisted laparoscopic colorectal surgery. Surg Clin North Am 83:1463–1468

22. Weber PA et al (2002) Telerobotic-assisted laparoscopic right and sigmoid colectomies for benign disease. Dis Colon Rectum 45:1689–1694; discussion 1695–1696

23. Munz Y et al (2004) Robotic assisted rectopexy. Am J Surg 187:88–92

24. Delaney CP et al (2003) Comparison of robotically performed and traditional laparoscopic colorectal surgery. Dis Colon Rectum 46:1633–1639

25. Gagner M, Lacroix A, Bolte E (1992) Laparoscopic adrenalectomy in Cushing's syndrome and pheochromocytoma. N Engl J Med 327:1033

26. Piazza L et al (1999) Laparoscopic robot-assisted right adrenalectomy and left ovariectomy (case reports). Chir Ital 51:465–466

27. Brunaud L et al (2003) [Advantages of using robotic Da Vinci system for unilateral adrenalectomy: early results]. Ann Chir 128:530–535

28. Lee BR et al (2000) Laparoscopic live donor nephrectomy: outcomes equivalent to open surgery. J Endourol 14:811–819; discussion 819–820

29. Ratner LE, Buell JF, Kuo PC (2000) Laparoscopic donor nephrectomy: pro. Transplantation 70:1544–1546

30. Schweitzer EJ et al (2000) Increased rates of donation with laparoscopic donor nephrectomy. Ann Surg 232:392–400

31. Horgan S et al (2002) Robotic-assisted laparoscopic donor nephrectomy for kidney transplantation. Transplantation 73:1474–1479

32. Buell JF et al (2002) Hand-assisted laparoscopic living-donor nephrectomy as an alternative to traditional laparoscopic living-donor nephrectomy. Am J Transplant 2:983–988

Evolving Endoluminal Therapies

10

Jeffrey L. Ponsky

While the past decade has seen the exciting growth of minimally invasive surgery through videoscopic technology, important advances have also been occurring in the area of endoluminal gastrointestinal therapy. In the past 30 years, the development of endoluminal gastrointestinal techniques has essentially revolutionized the treatment of colonic polyposis, peptic ulcer bleeding, choledocholithiasis, and the creation of enteral access for feeding. Other areas in which endoluminal therapy has had a great impact has been in the palliation of malignant obstruction of the biliary and gastrointestinal tracts by means of endoscopic stenting.

Laparoscopic approaches have established themselves as the gold standard for the treatment of gastroesophaeal reflux, morbid obesity, cholecystectomy, and appendectomy. Yet, new clinical and experimental work in flexible endoluminal and transluminal methodologies suggests that even less invasive procedures may be on the horizon.

10.1 Endoluminal Surgery

Initial endoscopic approaches to Barrett's esophagus have dealt with accurate diagnosis and staging of this condition. Early attempts at endoscopic ablation of Barrett's mucosa involved use of pinpoint thermal therapy and coagulation devices such as lasers, argon plasma coagulation, and bipolar probes. More recently photodynamic therapy has been utilized to destroy larger areas of abnormal mucosa. Attempts at endoscopic mucosal resection of larger areas of Barrett's mucosa have been accomplished and, as resection techniques become more refined, will undoubtedly replace ablation as the therapy of choice. The technique of endoscopic mucosal resection has been widely employed in Japan, and the method is rapidly being adopted throughout the world. This method has been applied to to the treatment of premalignant and superficial malignant lesions.

Endoscopic approaches to the therapy of gastroesophageal reflux are numerous and have led the way

in recent innovative application of new endoscopic technology. Endoscopic suturing was first described by Paul Swain. Devices based on his original design have been employed to place sutures at or near the esohagogastric junction in order to enhance the integrity of the lower esophageal sphincter and reduce reflux. The first device, EndoCinch (Bard) was used in a variety of clinical studies and offered initial promise of symptomatic improvement and reduction of consumed medication. It used a suction capsule design to grasp a bit of gastric wall and place a stitch. The mechanism was slow, inefficient, and a bit difficult to standardize. Unfortunately, little change was seen in objective criteria of reflux such as 24-h pH and esophageal manometry [1]. Third party payors were hesitant to compensate physicians and hospitals for these procedures, and use of the method has declined. Other technologies have attempted to approximate more closely the Nissen fundoplication by gathering tissue at the esophagogastric junction. The most visible of the latter is the Plicator device (NDO) [2]. The instrument is somewhat bulky and passed with an endoscope into the stomach. It is retroflexed and, under vision of the scope, gathers and sutures (full thickness) the tissue surrounding the gastric cardia. Although initial results are promising, no large series or long-term results are yet available for this procedure. It does, however, offer the durability of full-thickness gastric sutures with the promise of serosa to serosa healing.

Another developing endoluminal approach to gastroesophageal reflux is the injection of biopolymers into the submucosa or muscle of the esophageal wall, just above the esophagogastric junction [3]. Again, while promising and apparently quite easily performed, there are little available data regarding results. Perhaps one of the most attractive and well-studied therapies has been the application of radiofrequency energy into the esophageal wall by means of small needles mounted on an esophageal balloon (Stretta procedure). Energy is applied at numerous sites at six to eight levels around the esophagogastric junction. Early results suggested excellent relief of symptoms and high patient satisfaction. However, as in those with other aforementioned procedures, there were initially little objective data to support improvement. However, more recent studies involving evaluation of 24-h pH and manometry as well as a sham study seem to demonstrate documented reduction in reflux [4].

The mechanism by which the radiofrequency energy may work is thought to be twofold. Scarring in the distal esophageal wall may act as a barrier to reflux. In addition, there is some suggestion that vagal afferent fibers to the esophagus, which may normally produce transient relaxation of the distal sphincter, may destroyed by the thermal energy.

10.2 Transvisceral Surgery

Reports have emerged in the last few years of forays intothe new realm of transvisceral surgery. Investigators have endeavored to develop methods of endoscopically incising the stomach and passing a flexible endoscope into the peritoneal cavity where a variety of procedures have been attempted [5]. These have included gastrojejunostomy, fallopian tube ligation, appendectomy, and cholecystectomy. The organs removed are withdrawn through the stomach with the endoscope, and the gastric wall is sutured closed from within. Most of these procedures have been performed in animal models, but there are anecdotal reports in humans.

Clearly, the value and limits of such a concept will need to be defined. However, this new approach to intra-abdominal surgery is a new initiative in minimally invasive surgery. The incorporation of robotic manipulators to enhance complex maneuvers may also potentiate the value of these procedures.

While endoluminal endoscopic techniques have been deemed the realm of the gastroenterologist, they have continued to erode the domain of general surgeon with the development of effective and less invasive therapies for common disease processes. Surgeons will need to become involved in these methodologies or find themselves irrelevant in the future care of many common intra-abdominal maladies [6].

References

1. Chadalavada R, Lin E, Swafford V, Sedghi S, Smith CD (2004) Comparative results of endoluminal gastroplasty and laparoscopic antireflux surgery for the treatment of GERD. Surg Endosc 18:261–265

2. Chuttani R, Sud R, Sachdev G, Puri R, Kozarek R, Haber G, Pleskow D, Zaman M, Lembo A (2003) A novel endoscopic full-thickness plcator for the treatment of GERD: a pilot study. Gastrointest Endosc 58:770–776

3. Edmundowicz SA (2004) Injection therapy of the lower esophageal sphincter for the treatment of GERD. Gastrointest Endosc 59:545–552

4. Triadafilopoulos G (2004) Changes in GERD symptom scores correlate with improvement in esophageal acid exposure after the Stretta procedure. Surg Endosc 18:1038–1044

5. Kalloo AN, Singh VK, Jagannath SB, Niiyama H, Hill SL, Vaughn CA, Magee CA, Kantsevoy SV (2004) Flexible transgastric peritoneoscopy: A novel approach to diagnostic and therapeutic interventions in the peritoneal cavity. Gastrointest Endosc 60:114–117

6. Chand B, Felsher J, Ponsky JL (2003) Future trends in flexible endoscopy. Semin Laparosc Surg 10:49–54

Part IV
Innovations in Surgical Instruments

Microtechnology in Surgical Devices

11

Marc O. Schurr

11.1 Introduction

Microtechnology plays an important role in the development of medical and surgical devices. Since the early 1990s [13], there has been growing interest in using microtechnology for miniaturization of medical devices or for increasing their functionality through the integration of smart components and sensors.

Microsystems technology (MST), as it is called in Europe, or microelectromechanical systems (MEMS), as it is called in the United States, combine electronic with mechanical components at a very high level of systems integration. Microsystems are smart devices that integrate sensors, actuators, and intelligent electronics for on-board signal processing [27]. In the industrial area these technologies are used to make various kinds of sensor elements, such as accelerometers for airbags in cars, microfluidic components, such as inkjet print heads, and other elements. In the medical field, MST is used in a number of products such as pacemakers or hearing implants [5]. While most MST components are produced using semiconductor processes [27], there are a number of alternative technologies enabling the production of a broad variety of microdevices and components in virtually all industry sectors. The potential of MST for medical use was recognized more than a decade ago [13, 14], and has since then led to the development of numerous practical applications [21].

Sometimes MST and nanotechnology are terms that are used synonymously since both concern miniaturized devices. However, both technologies are entirely different. While MST deals with components in the submillimeter size, nanotechnology concerns submicrometer structures. Nanotechnology mainly refers to innovating material properties such as nanostructured surfaces with special biocompatibility features and may be an important enabler for future biomedical products in the future, also combined with MST devices.

Based on the high density of functional integration and the small space requirements, MST components are enhancing surgical devices in different areas, and can be subdivided into the following applications:

- Extracorporeal devices such as telemetric health monitoring systems (e.g., wearable electrocardiogram [ECG] monitors)
- Intracorporeal devices such as intelligent surgical instruments (e.g., tactile laparoscopic instruments)
- Implantable devices such as telemetric implants (e.g., cardiac pacemakers)
- Endoscopic diagnostic and interventional systems such as telemetric capsule endoscopes

Recently there has been an increase in medical MST-related research and development (R&D) activities, both on the side of research institutes and industry. While routine clinical applications of MST-enhanced surgical devices are still limited to a number of larger volume applications such as pacemakers [28] (Fig. 11.1), a number of developments are in later-stage experimental research or in clinical studies. Medical applications of MST technologies are growing at double-digit compounded growth rates [17], which led to a forecasted global market volume of over $ 1 billion in 2006.

11.2 MST in Medical Devices: Challenges and Opportunities

The community developing and using MST for medical devices is a very heterogeneous scene of academic researchers, specialized MST companies, medical device corporations, start-ups, and clinicians. In order to better understand the challenges and opportunities of MST in medical devices, our institute has a conducted global survey among executives from research and industry on the use of medical microsystems technology. This survey was done in 2004 within the scope of the netMED project funded by the European Union (GIRT-CT-2002-05113). The study was based on a standardized questionnaire and included 110 persons, with about 50% of participants coming from the medical device industry and the remaining participants from R&D institutes and MST companies.

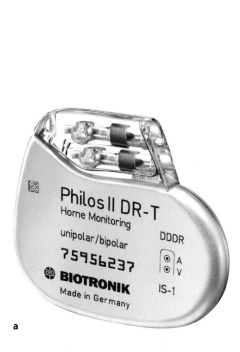

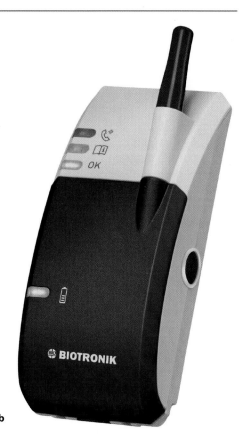

a

b

Fig. 11.1 Telemetric pacemaker for remote patient monitoring. Source: Biotronik GmbH, Berlin, Germany. **a** Pacemaker with telemetry units. **b** Mobile data transfer unit, like a cellular phone

Asked about the advantages expected in the next 5 years from the applications of MST in medical devices, the study participants named new product opportunities for existing market segments and for entering new market segments along with product miniaturization potential as their key expectation. The most important barriers to innovation in medical MST are high initial investment load, general skepticism of users (doctors, patients), and unclear reimbursement conditions for MST-enhanced medical devices or MST-related diagnostic or therapeutic procedures. This mainly refers to telemetric technologies such as remote ECG diagnostics and remote cardiac pacemaker or implantable defibrillator monitoring.

Asked about the preconditions necessary to improve the application of MST in medical devices, survey participants named the availability of standardized MST elements, comparable to standardized electronic elements, customizable integrated systems to facilitate the use of MST components in medical devices, and the increase of acceptance of these technologies among payers in the health care system.

This shows that barriers to innovation in the field of medical MST are not only on the side of the technology with its particular challenges, but also on the market side in terms of unsolved issues in medical high-tech reimbursement. This applies especially to the European market place.

As for the types of microsystems components judged most important for medical products in the future, our study participants named various types of sensors such as biosensors, chemical sensors, pressure sensors, and microfluidic structures. This indicates that experts see the future of MST in medical devices mainly in the improvement of device intelligence through sensors and in using microactuators for miniaturization intervention instruments (Fig. 11.2).

Of particular importance will be the definition of standards [15] and common interfaces to facilitate the use of MST components, especially in markets with smaller product volumes, such as medicine, if compared with large-scale industrial applications, such as automotive, environmental of aerospace.

11.3 Areas of MST Applications in Medical Devices

As mentioned above, the application of MST components in medical devices can mainly be grouped into four different areas. This classification refers to current

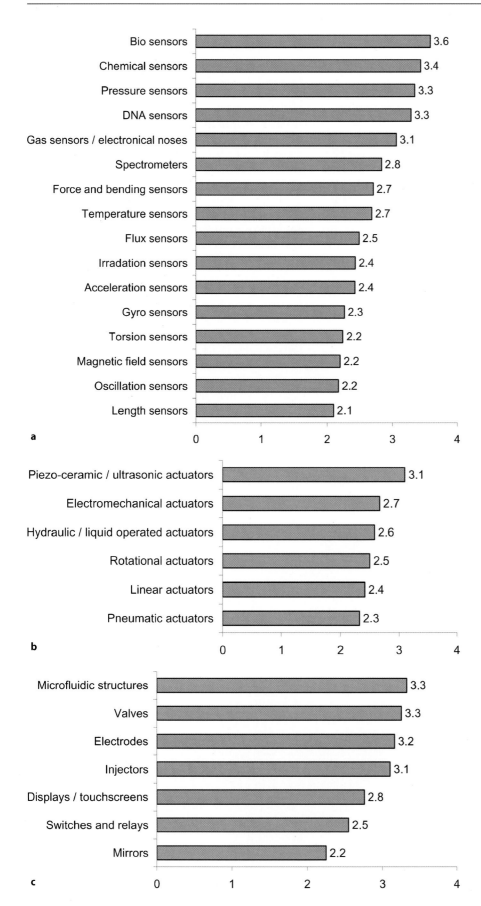

Fig. 11.2 netMED global survey on medical microsystems technology: types of microsystems components seen most important for medical products in the future. **a** Sensors. **b** Actuators. **c** Other

focal applications of MST in the medical field and is neither systematic nor complete.

11.3.1 Extracorporeal MST-Enhanced Devices

The area of extracorporeal MST-enhanced devices is probably the most mature and established field of MST applications. There are numerous examples of MST components integrated into external diagnostic and monitoring systems. These include handheld diagnostic devices such as optical bilirubin analyzers based on a MST spectrometer [29], sensors embedded into smart textiles or wearable ECG foils [2] (Fig. 11.3).

Often MST applications are combined with wireless technologies to enable patient monitoring without restrictions in mobility. Miniaturized telemetry units using the Bluetooth standard transmit parameters to a patient data management systems and electronic patient records. This allows both the patient and the attending physician to deal efficiently with monitoring data.

11.3.2 Intracorporeal MST-Enhanced Devices

Intracorporeal but not implantable medical and surgical devices use MST components to provide additional qualities and functions that cannot be realized with

standard technology. A good example of this class of MST applications is sensor-enhanced surgical instruments. The concept of restoring tactile feedback in laparoscopic surgery has been around for more than a decade. Several attempts have been made to integrate tactile sensors into the jaws of laparoscopic instruments to allow palpation and mechanical characterization of tissues during surgery, such as the surgeon would do with his or her hand in open surgery [22]. In the past, some attempts to create tactile sensors have failed, partly related to complex technologies that could not be efficiently applied in this small market segment.

Since tactile sensing in laparoscopic surgery is still an attractive proposition from a medical standpoint, new attempts are being made to realize such instruments on a more cost-friendly technology basis.

One of these is a program carried out by our own institution to develop a polymer sensor array, which is elastic, compliant and can be attached to the tip of a laparoscopic instrument as a disposable. This sensor (Fig. 11.4) is composed of a conductive and a resistive layer of polymer separated by a perforated layer.

Through exerting external pressure, the resistive coupling between the elastic conductive membranes is changed, indicating the force across the sensor array. The current forceps prototype (Fig. 11.5) has an array with 32 sensory elements. The force exerted on each element is visualized on a display. Experimental evaluation of the tactile forceps has shown that objects of different size and hardness can be well different shaded from their neighboring structures.

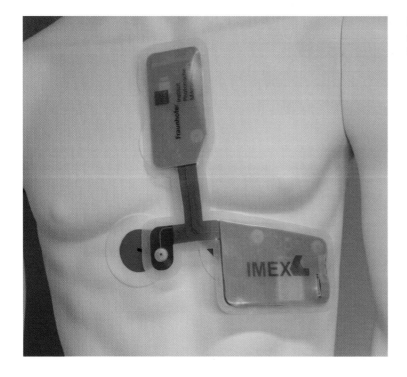

Fig. 11.3 Telemetric three-channel ECG system. Source: Fraunhofer Institute Photonic Microsystems, Dresden, Germany

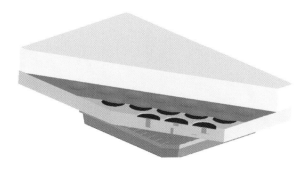

Fig. 11.4 A polymer microsensor for tactile laparoscopic instruments (schematic drawing)

In animal experiments (Fig. 11.6) objects simulating lymph nodes at the mesenteric root could be localized and differentiated using the instrument.

Further research will be required to optimize the sensitivity and the applicability of tactile sensor arrays for laparoscopic surgery.

Another example of intracorporeal MST applications is advanced optical diagnostic systems for microscopic analysis of tissues in situ [7]. The concept of confocal laser scanning microscopy is widely known in the histological examination of tissues samples. Using the miniaturization potential of MST, laser scanning microscopes can be scaled down to a level that they can be used via an endoscope directly inside the human body, e.g., for in situ analysis of lesions suspicious for cancer [8]. Figure 11.7 shows a prototype two axes microscanner with two miniature mirrors etched from silicon, compared with the size of a regular 10-mm laparoscope. The two electrostatically driven mirrors pivot and scan the laser beam across the tissue surface at video speed.

The resulting fluorescence can be enhanced by local tissue staining techniques. Figure 11.8 compares histological images obtained by this fluorescence laser scanning microscopy technique with conventional hematoxylin and eosin (HE)-stained histology.

11.3.3 Implantable MST Devices

Telemetric implants are among the most important applications of MST in medicine. MST components implanted into the human body include sensors of various types that measure specific health parameters, such as blood glucose [18] or blood pressure or flow [1, 4, 30]. The signals are then transferred via telemetric coils to readout device outside of the body. A good example for existing products in this field is cardiac pacemakers or defibrillators that are equipped with miniaturized telemetry units to send cardiac parameters and parameters or their electrical interaction with a heart outside of the body [28] (Fig. 11.1). The data are received by a readout device similar to a cellular GSM phone and then sent from there to a remote cardiovascular service center.

This allows improvement of patient monitoring and implant maintenance, without the need to see the patient regularly. These kinds of telemetrically enhanced cardiovascular implants based on MST are available on the market for clinical use; in addition to the product, advanced cardiovascular monitoring services are provided by the same manufacturer.

Other applications of intracorporeal MST include the use of telemetric sensors for diagnostic and disease monitoring purposes. Examples include the measure-

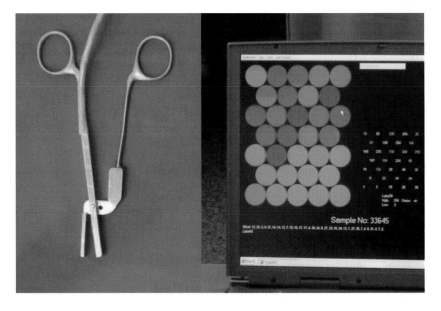

Fig. 11.5 A prototype of a tactile surgical instrument with the polymer sensor and force display system

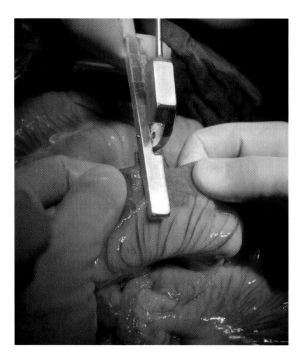

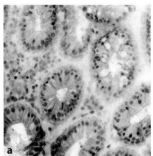

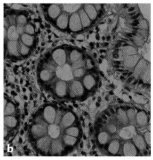

Fig. 11.6 Palpating an object simulating a lymph node at the mesenteric root (animal experiment)

Fig. 11.8 Histological images obtained by fluorescence laser scanning microscopy technique (**a**), with conventional HE-stained histology (**b**). This experimental program has been conducted by a group of several research institutes, supported by grants from BMBF, Germany, and the European Union

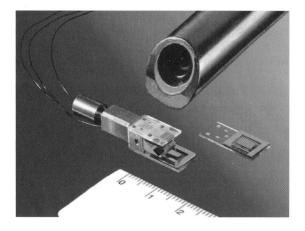

Fig. 11.7 Microscanner for confocal fluorescence microscopy. Source: Medea Project, supported by the European Union

comprises several MST components such as a pressure sensor and miniaturized telemetry coils. The medical concept behind this device is to monitor blood pressure values and to better adjust antihypertensive medication in order to reach normal blood pressure values in a higher number of patients. Today only in a minority of patients normotensive blood pressure values are achieved due to a lack in adequate monitoring and patient management means.

This example underlines the principle that implantable sensory MST devices are mainly targeting secondary disease prevention by slowing down disease progression or avoiding complications through consequent and consistent monitoring. Thus, MST-based monitoring systems will may a major impact on the prevention of disease progression to the benefit of both the patient and the healthcare system.

Also on the therapeutic side, MST applications are important sources of innovation. Specific implants have been equipped with microsensors in order to monitor the function of the implant. Examples of this kind of application of MST in surgery include pressure sensors integrated into endovascular stent grafts in order to detect residual blood flow through the aneurysm sac in endovascular treatment of abdominal aortic aneu-

ment of intravesical pressure in paraplegic persons to avoid overfilling of the bladder and the urinary tract [6].

Our own group has been working with the company Sensocor, Ltd., Karlsruhe, Germany, in the development of an implantable telemetric blood pressure measurement sensor for the monitoring of hypertension (Fig. 11.9). The implant is an integrated device that

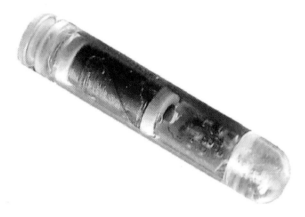

Fig. 11.9 Concept of an implantable blood pressure measurement. Source: Sensocor, Ltd., Karlsruhe, Germany. The implant is an integrated device that comprises several MST components such as pressure sensors and miniaturized telemetry coils

rysm [3]. Another approach is to use microsensors in implants to detect concomitant disease, such as detection of glaucoma through pressure sensors integrated into an intraocular lens graft implanted for the treatment of cataract [26].

Also, the field of replacing lost organ function, and organ stimulation MST-based implants are of interest. This includes the restoration of lost or impaired sensory functions of the ear [5] and the eye [12, 20], or of traumatized nerves [23–25].

11.3.4 MST in Endoscopy

The field of endoscopy is an interesting area for the application of MST, since high-functional integration and miniaturization, the two main characteristics of MST, are an important advantage in this field.

Besides microfiberoptics for the inspection of smallest tubular organs and body cavities, a big interest is in using MST for creating new locomotion technologies in the human body. A very good example is capsule endoscopy [9] using a miniaturized optical camera system with telemetric image data transfer integrated into an ingestible capsule. A number of MST elements are used to realize the Pill-Cam capsule endoscope of Given Imaging, Ltd., Yoqneam, Israel, such as CMOS image sensors, LED illumination diodes, imaging electronics, and telemetric signal transfer components.

Farther down the road are self-locomoting endoscopes that, unlike a capsule endoscope, can actively propel through the digestive organs and be steered into the desired direction. A good example for this

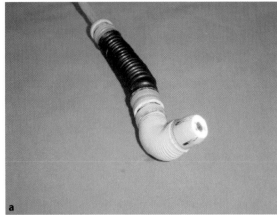

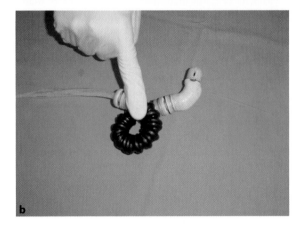

Fig. 11.10 The E^2 self-propelling endoscope is a pneumatically controlled inchworm that moves through the colon by a sequential adhering to the bowel wall and elongating/shortening the midsection. **a** Inchworm with imaging head and propelling body. **b** High flexibility

class of MST applications is the E^2 endoscope system of Era Endoscopy Srl, Pontedera, Italy, based on research [16] conducted by the CRIM laboratory of Scuola Superiore Sant'Anna, Pisa (supported by a grant of IMC/KIST, Seoul, South Korea). The E^2 self-propelling endoscope (Fig. 11.10) is a pneumatically controlled inchworm that moves through the colon by sequentially adhering to the bowel wall with its proximal and its distal end and elongating/shortening the midsection.

The MST components used for this technology besides the CMOS imaging and LED illumination include microfluidic and -filter elements to support the pneumatic locomotion mechanism. The clinical purpose behind self-propelling microendoscopes lies in the reduction of the force exerted to the tissue, thus the reduction of pain during the procedure. The clinical benefit will be improved patient acceptance of colonoscopy cancer screening programs in the future.

11.4   Discussion

Microsystems technology is nowadays playing a major role for improving products in the health care sector. In the last years, the development of MST applications has been boosted by the ability to manufacture MST elements with high precision, reliability, and at acceptable costs. A considerable number of products used in clinical routine today are functionally based on MST and allied technologies.

These applications include the medical high volume markets of cardiac rhythm management [28] or implantable hearing aids [5], as well as highly specialized applications in the field of neural rehabilitation [23].

Rebello [17] has identified a minimum of 25 major research programs internationally, focusing only on surgical MST and surgical sensors. This shows there are major research efforts in progress that will deliver further leads for device companies to develop advanced medical products on the basis of MST.

The world market projection for MST and MST components in medical products was expected to exceed $1 billion by 2005 or 2006. This considerable market potential will attract more industrial players to invest into microtechnology for medical and surgical products.

The clinical foundation for promoting the use of MST in medicine is mainly based on the significant potential of MST to enable products that improve early disease detection and the monitoring of chronic illnesses. This refers to a number of the most important health problems such as cardiovascular disease, hypertension, diabetes, and cancer, to name just a few. The possibility to provide better diagnostic techniques based on microstructures, such as confocal fluorescence microscopy [8] may significantly improve the efficiency of early cancer detection programs.

Besides the future advantages for the diagnostic precision and diagnostic quality, MST can also deliver advantages directly to the patient. In the field of self-propelled endoscopy [16], MST components play an important role in reducing the forces that are exerted to the tissue. The reduction of force will directly address pain and discomfort during cancer screening colonoscopy, thus improving the willingness of individuals to attend a cancer prevention program.

In addition to the significant opportunities that MST brings for innovating medical devices, there are also several particular challenges that need to be addressed. One of the key hurdles for using MST more widely in medical products is the enormous cost involved into the development and the design of MST components. In large industrial applications, this cost is offset against high production volumes. In many specialized medical applications, however, production volumes are relatively small compared with industrial dimensions.

Increasing standardization of MST components may help to solve this problem. Similar to electronics, where well-defined standardized components are available at low cost, standardized MST components such as pressure sensors, telemetry units, or optical structures not dedicated to a single application but for multiple purposes will become available. To achieve this goal, it is important to formulate and respect technical standards [15].

But there are also a number of nontechnical problems for MST that need to be overcome. Among the most important barriers to innovation seen by specialists from the field are unclear reimbursement conditions [10]. This shows that the further progress MST in medicine not only depends on successful R&D and the establishment of technical standards, but also on the availability of innovative reimbursement schemes that act as incentives for the use of advanced technology, particularly in the areas of disease prevention and early detection. Especially in these fields can innovation provide a significant leverage on reducing healthcare costs in the mid and long term. This needs to be reflected in reimbursement for medical care enabled by MST or other advanced technologies.

References

1. Clasbrummel B, Muhr G, Moellenhoff G (2004) Pressure sensors for the monitoring of diseases in surgical care. Min Invas Ther Allied Technol 13:105–109

2. Despang G, Holland HJ, Fischer WJ, Marschner U, Boden R (2004) Bluetooth body area network für TeleHomeCare-Anwendungen. Biomed Tech 49(Suppl):250–251

3. Ellozy SH, Carroccio A, Lookstein RA, Minor ME, Sheahan CM, Juta J, Cha A, Valenzuela R, Addis MD, Jacobs TS, Teodorescu VJ, Marin ML (2004) First experience in human beings with a permanently implantable intrasac pressure transducer for monitoring endovascular repair of abdominal aortic aneurysms. J Vasc Surg 40:405–412

4. Ericson MN, Wilson MA Cote GL, Baba JS, Xu W, Bobrek CL, Hileman MS, Emery MS, Lenarduzzi R (2004) Implantable sensor for blood flow monitoring after transplant surgery. Min Invas Ther Allied Technol 13:87–94

5. Federspil PA, Plinkert PK (2004) Restoring hearing with active hearing implants. Biomed Tech (Berl) 49:78–82

6. Fischer H, Haller D, Echtle D (2002) Minimally invasive pressure sensor for telemetric recording of intravesical pressure in the human. Biomed Tech (Berl) 47(Suppl 1):338–341

7. George M (2004) optical methods and sensors for in situ histology and endoscopy. Min Invas Ther Allied Technol 13:95–104

8. George M, Albrecht HJ, Schurr MO, Papageorgas P, Hofmann U, Maroulis D, Depeursinge C, Iakkovidis D, Theofanous N, Menciassi A (2003) A laser-scanning endoscope base on monosilicon micromachined mirrors with enhanced attributes. Novel Optical Instrumentation for Biomedical Applications Proc. SPIE, vol. 2003:5143

9. Gong F, Swain P, Mills T. (2000) Wireless endoscopy. Gastrointest Endosc 51:725–729

10. Kalanovic D, Schurr MO (2004) Innovation requirements for telemetric sensor systems in medicine: results of a survey in Germany. Min Invas Ther Allied Technol 13:68–77

12. Laube T, Schanze T, Brockmann C, Bolle I, Stieglitz T, Bornfeld N (2003) Chronically implanted epidural electrodes in Gottinger minipigs allow function tests of epiretinal implants. Graefes Arch Clin Exp Ophthalmol 241:1013–1019

13. Menz W, Buess G (1993) Potential applications of microsystems engineering in minimal invasive surgery. Endosc Surg Allied Technol 1:171–180

14. Menz W, Guber A (1994) Microstructure technologies and their potential in medical applications. Minim Invasive Neurosurg 1994 37:21–27

15. Neuder K, Dehm J (2004) Technical standards for microsensors in surgery and minimally invasive therapy. Min Invas Ther Allied Technol 13:110–113

16. Phee L, Accoto D, Menciassi A, Stefanini C, Carrozza MC, Dario P (2002) Analysis and development of locomotion devices for the gastrointestinal tract. IEEE Trans Biomed Eng 49:613–616

17. Rebello K (2004) Applications of MEMS in surgery. Proc IEEE 92:1

18. Renard E (2004) Implantable glucose sensors for diabetes monitoring. Min Invas Ther Allied Technol 13:78–86

19. Renard E (2004) Implantable insulin delivery pumps. Min Invas Ther Allied Technol 13:328–335

20. Sachs HG, Gabel VP Retinal replacement—the development of microelectronic retinal prostheses—experience with subretinal implants and new aspects. Graefes Arch Clin Exp Ophthalmol 242:717–723

21. Schurr MO (2004) Sensors in minimally invasive therapy – a technology coming of age. Invas Ther Allied Technol 13:67

22. Schurr MO, Heyn SP, Menz W, Buess G (1998) Endosystems – future perspectives for endoluminal therapy. Min Invas Ther Allied Technol 13:37–42

23. Stieglitz T (2002) Implantable microsystems for monitoring and neural rehabilitation, part II. Med Device Technol 13:24–27

24. Stieglitz T, Meyer JU (1999) Implantable microsystems. Polyimide-based neuroprostheses for interfacing nerves. Med Device Technol :28–30

25. Stieglitz T, Schuettler M, Koch KP (2004) Neural prostheses in clinical applications—trends from precision mechanics towards biomedical microsystems in neurological rehabilitation. Biomed Tech (Berl) 49:72–77

26. Svedbergh B, Backlund Y, Hok B, Rosengren L The IOP-IOL. A probe into the eye. Acta Ophthalmol (Copenh) 70:266–268

27. Wagner B (1995) Principles of development and design of microsystems. Endosc Surg Allied Technol 3:204–209

28. Wildau HJ (2004) Wireless remote monitoring for patients with atrial tachyarrhythmias. J Electrocardiol 37(Suppl):53–54

29. Wong CM, van Dijk PJ, Laing IA (2002) A comparison of transcutaneous bilirubinometers: SpectRx BiliCheck versus Minolta AirShields. Arch Dis Child Fetal Neonatal Ed 87:F137–F40

30. Zacheja J, Wenzel D, Bach T, Clasbrummel B (1998) Micromechanical pressure sensors for medical evaluation of blood vessels and bypasses after surgical intervention. Biomed Tech (Berl) 43(Suppl):182–183

Innovative Instruments in Endoscopic Surgery

12

Gerhard F. Bueß and Masahiro Waseda

12.1 Introduction

Endoscopic surgery has conditions that are different from open surgery, insofar as the need for specific instrument design exists. Instruments for endoscopic surgery are introduced through round trocars with round seals, which means that they are basically always constructed in form of tube-like structures, allowing gastight sealing when the instruments are introduced [1].

Further specific conditions exist because of the limited degrees of freedom [2] when an instrument is introduced through a normal trocar sleeve. This means, for example, that needles for sutures cannot be guided in the optimal way. The conditions for the placement of endoscopic instruments often result in a nonergonomic working position so that the surgeon does not have optimal conditions for the work. Compared with open surgery, the possibility of using ligatures to transect vessel guiding structures is limited, as is the possibility of achieving hemostasis when bleeding occurs.

An increasingly important part of endoscopic surgery is endoluminal surgery. In addition to the points abovementioned in endoluminal surgery, for example in the rectum cavity, we are forced to work in a small working space, and the ability to introduce different instruments at the same time is limited because of the small space and the limited access [3].

12.2 Innovative Instruments for Laparoscopic Surgery

12.2.1 Curved Instruments

The possibility of reaching optimal working conditions is restricted by the use of straight instruments. We started in 1980 to develop instruments for endorectal surgery, and we noticed that curves and bayonet-formed angulations brought significant advantages in the maneuverability of the instruments (see below). The use of optimal curves in instrument design allows,

for example, an optimal placement of a needle and modification of the direction of the needle [4].

A needle holder and suture grasper design has been developed by the Wolf Company [5], which gives an ideal advantage in directing the position of the needle in the needle holder. Figure 12.1 shows the suture of the fundic wrap. The round needle holder allows optimal positioning of the needle, and the golden tip of the suture grasper always gives the best view to the tip of the needle and provides the best possible conditions to manipulate the needle (Fig. 12.2).

Instruments with larger curves have to be introduced through a flexible trocar. Figure 12.3 shows the curved window grasper and the flexible trocar. Figure 12.4 shows the introduction of the curved window grasper through the flexible trocar. The intra-abdominal situation of the curved instrument is demonstrated in Figure 12.5: The curved instrument has a number of advantages during surgical manipulation. The most important advantage is better ergonomic position, which

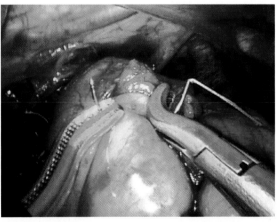

Fig. 12.1 Suture of the fundic wrap. The needle holder on the *right side* is driving the needle; the suture grasper with the golden tip is holding the tip of the needle. The curve of the suture grasper gives optimal view of the needle and a good hold in all different positions

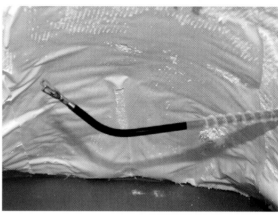

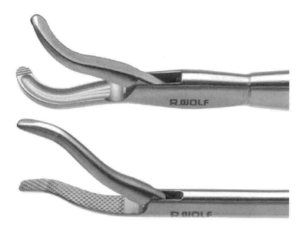

Fig. 12.2 Needle holder (*upper half* of the image) and suture grasper (*lower half* of the image). The needle holder gives a firm hold on the needle in different positions. The tip of the needle holder has an atraumatic area for grasping the suture. The suture grasper has a uniform profile, so that the needle can be held strongly enough, and the suture material is not destroyed by the surface

Fig. 12.5 Curved window grasper introduced through the flexible trocar and simulation of the abdominal wall

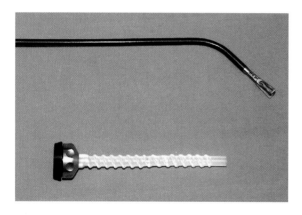

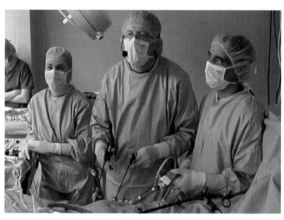

Fig. 12.3 Curved window grasper (*upper half*) and a flexible trocar

Fig. 12.6 Ergonomical working position for the surgeon by the use of a curved instrument. Both working instruments of the surgeon are on the right side of optic, so that there is no conflict with the camera assistant

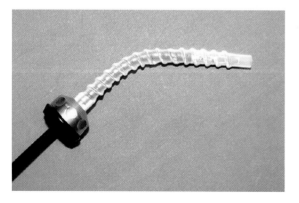

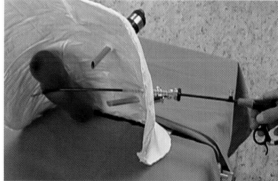

Fig. 12.4 Introduction of the instrument through the flexible trocar

Fig. 12.7 Demonstration of retraction by the use of the back of the curved instrument. The curve is less traumatic when compared with the tip of a straight instrument

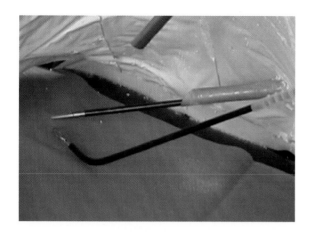

Fig. 12.8 Demonstration of the angle between the curved and the straight instrument. Although the two instruments are close together and in parallel position, there is an optimal working angle between them

is demonstrated in Figure 12.6: The curved instrument allows an assistant guiding the camera at the side of the surgeon. The instruments of the surgeon are in a parallel position because of the advantage of the angulation of the instrument tip.

Better retraction is possible by the use of the curve of the instrument shown in Figure 12.7. The angle between the two working instruments due to the angulation is demonstrated in Figure 12.8. Only this condition affords the surgeon a convenient ergonomic parallel working position of the hands and an optimal working angle between the instruments themselves.

An additional advantage of the curves is the possibility to encircle structures, for example the esophagus in fundoplication [6]. In case of mechanical conflict between instruments, only the rotation of the curved instrument has to be changed to allow again free handling of the endoscopic instrumentation.

12.2.2 Instruments with All Degrees of Freedom for Suturing: the Radius Surgical System

Following early experience with conventional endoscopic suturing systems, we began with the research center in Karlsruhe, Germany, in the development of instruments with all degrees of freedom [7]. In the early 1990s, we could already perform experimental tests with the use of angulating instruments that could turn at the tip. In the following years, we developed the first robotic systems for endoscopic surgery, and performed the first animal experiments and distant operations [8].

The application of robotic systems in endoscopic surgery demonstrates that this technology is highly complex and expensive, and that only few hospitals succeeded to integrate the robotic systems into routine surgery on an economical acceptable basis [7]. We therefore decided to start our own company, Tübingen Scientific [9], with a program to develop a suturing system with intuitive and ergonomic handling that allows deflection and rotation of the tip of the instruments so that comparable free placement of the direction of suture is given as in the use of robotic systems. Figure 12.9 demonstrates the place of the radius surgical

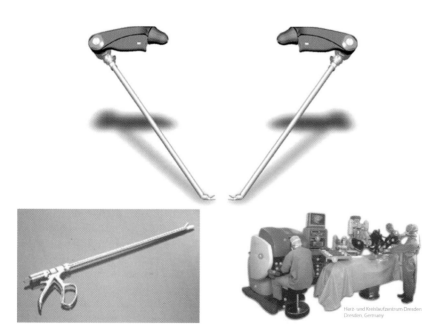

Fig. 12.9 The radius surgical system between conventional instruments and robotics. This system allows deflection of the tip and rotation of the tip in a deflected position. A specific new handle design is necessary to enhanced the degrees of freedom

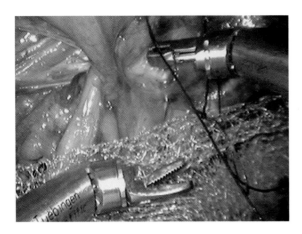

Fig. 12.10 Suture of a mesh to the inguinal ligament using the degrees of freedom afforded by the radius system

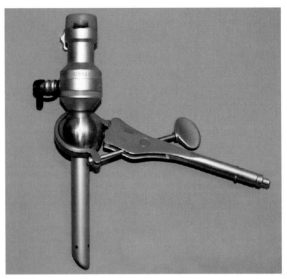

Fig. 12.11 The ball trocar of the endofreeze system. The ball represents the invariant point for turning the instrument. One screw at the trocar shaft and one at the metal ring allow adjustment for the friction of movement

system between conventional instruments and robotic systems. This can also be defined as a mechanical manipulator. When the handle of the system is brought forward, the tip is straight; when the handle is flexed to 45°, the tip of the instrument is flexed to a 70° position. Rotation of the tip is accomplished by rotating the knob at the tip of the handle. Complete rotation of the instrument tip is in this way possible. The whole system can be completely dismantled and cleaned without problem. One of the most important applications of the suturing system in our hands is in the moment the suturing of meshes to the abdominal wall to the inguinal ligament in case of an inguinal hernia.

In this way, we have for the first time enabled the ability to perform a precise suture inside the abdomen for optimal mesh fixation. Experiments [10, 11] have demonstrated that the preciseness of the stitches is much higher and the strength of the stitches is stronger compared with sutures using conventional needle drivers. Figure 12.10 demonstrates the suturing of a mesh with the use of radius.

12.2.3 The Endofreeze System

This system is designed to perform solo surgery. It is a very simple construction, which allows one to hold the camera or to hold retracting instruments. The position of camera or instruments can be changed against a cer-

tain friction with only one hand, and it stays automatically in the new position.

Figure 12.11 shows the ball trocar. The system itself was developed by Tübingen Scientific, and production and marketing is performed by Aesculap [12]. The ball trocar has always to be inserted until the ball touches the abdominal wall to achieve a good position of the invariant point. The screw at the shaft of the trocar and the screw at the metal ring holding the ball allow an adjustment of the friction so that a movement to a new position is possible with the use of only one hand, and that the new position is kept stabile by the optimal defined friction.

Figure 12.12 shows the routine application of solo surgery in cholecystectomy. The camera and the retracting forceps are held by two ball trocars, linked to the operative table by a Leila retractor (Aesculap). With the right hand, the surgeon is guiding a combination instrument, with the left hand, the curved grasper that again, allows an optimal ergonomic working position and a good angle inside the abdomen between the tips of the instruments. Setup and positioning time by the use of Endofreeze both with the use of a Leila or Unitrac retractor comes close to the time needed in a conventional control group. They are clearly faster than any other advanced electronic camera-guiding systems [13]. Endofreeze in a way similar to the radius system fulfilled the task—to have simple tools available that are not too expensive, so that they can easily be used in routine surgery.

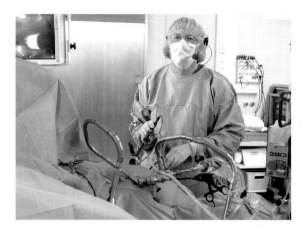

Fig. 12.12 Solo surgery of a cholecystectomy with the use of two endofreeze systems. On the right side of the patient a 5-mm instrument for retraction of the gallbladder. At the umbilicus is a 10-mm ball trocar for holding the camera. Ergonomic working position of the surgeon due to the use of a curved window grasper

12.2.4 Combination Instruments for Endoscopic Surgery

With a routine laparoscopic cholecystectomy, we prefer the combination of blunt and sharp dissection when the gallbladder is dissected. To avoid the need for instrument changes, we have designed a combination instrument that allows the integration of a hook for dissection [1]. When the hook is pulled backward into the shaft, blunt dissection is possible; when the hook is moved forward, a sharp dissection with high frequency can be performed easily.

Figure 12.13 demonstrates the function of rinsing and suction using the laparoscopic combination instrument.

12.3 Endoluminal Surgery of Rectum and Colon

The first endoscopic procedure for the rectal cavity was designed in 1980 [14] and has been in clinical application for more than 22 years. Figure 12.14 demonstrates the principle of the procedure [15]: Stereoscopic optic gives optimal view, gas dilatation allows good exposition of the rectal cavity, and the curved instruments allow a better access in typical positions of the tumor, so that optimal surgical performance is given.

This image with the three instruments also demonstrates the problem of integrating three instruments. When the active instruments of the surgeon are moved, they often collide with a third instrument, which normally is the suction device. Another disadvantage of this technique is that to prevent a collision, the suction device is often pulled backward and is therefore out of view. In this position, the suction device cannot remove the smoke from the cavity, so that the quality of view is diminished.

Together with ERBE (Tübingen, Germany), we have designed a highly complex combination instrument. This instrument by ERBE [16] has a specific design (Fig. 12.15): The curves at the tip allow optimal access to the area of the rectal wall and perirectal space. The curve close to the handle is necessary to prevent conflicts with optic and other instrument handles.

The instrument does include four different main functions: a needle for cutting; in the upper tube (dem-

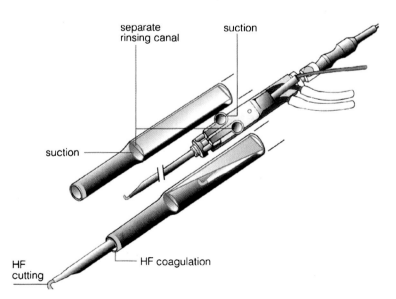

Fig. 12.13 A graphical demonstration of the Wolf combination instruments. Rinsing, suction, and coagulation by the tip are possible by the outer sheath of the combination instrument. The integrated hook allows sharp dissection. The tip can be pulled backward into the shaft of the combination instrument for unrestricted rinsing, suction, and coagulation

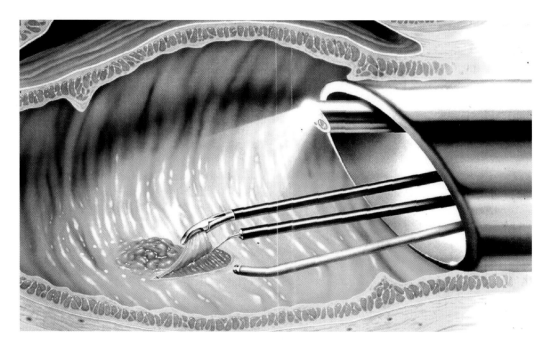

Fig. 12.14 The instrumentation for transanal endoscopic microsurgery (TEM) introduced into the rectal cavity; stereoscopic optic view above gives optimal view. Three curved instruments used in this application

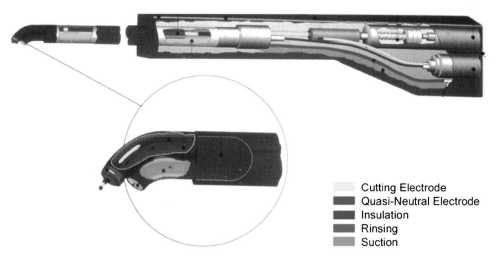

Cutting Electrode
Quasi-Neutral Electrode
Insulation
Rinsing
Suction

Fig. 12.15 TEM-Erbe combination instrument. Through the upper tube the cutting needle can be pushed forward and backward. The tip of the upper tube allows coagulation, the lower tube suction

onstrated in blue) the channel for rinsing; at the tip of the upper tube a metal ring for coagulation; and in the lower tube a suction channel for the removal of fluids and smoke.

When cutting is performed, the needle has to be pushed forward; for coagulation, it must be pulled backward into the lumen. This task is completed by an electronic controlled pneumatic drive. When the yellow foot pedal is pressed, the pneumatic pushes the needle forward. When coagulation is activated or when for a short period no activation of the cutting electrode is performed, the needle is automatically pulled backward.

As in many situations, the combination does not only add different functions, but also giveesclear additional advantages. The fact that no change of instrument is necessary allows in the case of a bleeder no time loss, and suction is quickly possible, as is coagulation [17]. At the same time, the smoke generated by cutting or coagulation is automatically removed at the tip of the instrument, so the view during dissection is much better.

The combination instrument allows that during all the TEM procedure it is never necessary to use more than two instruments, which gives much more freedom in movement and as mentioned above, clear additional advantages. These advantages are specifically important in endoluminal surgery, where the lumen of the organ is restricting significantly the possibility to introduce additional instruments.

12.4 Full-Thickness Resection Device, the Concept of a New Device for Removal of Polyps from the Rectum and Descending Colon

More than 20 years ago, we worked on the design of a semicircular stapler, to be introduced into the TEM instrument [18]. The idea of this concept was to make full-thickness resections as simple as possible and to reduce possible complications by opening the perirectal spaces.

Years later, we were approached by Boston Scientific [19] with the aim to jointly develop a stapling device that allows full-thickness resection. After a long development period, we had the chance for experimental evaluation of a short and a long version of the new full-thickness resection device (FTRD). This device (Fig. 12.16) consists of a handle, which allows the insertion of two graspers, and a thin-lumen flexible endoscope. Attached is a flexible shaft with two different lengths, which allow either to reach the rectosigmoid junction or the splenic flexure. Into the head is integrated a resection chamber that includes a semicircular stapler for resection of full-thickness parts of the bowel.

Under the endoscopic view of the flexible endoscope, the healthy wall beside the tumor is grasped with special retraction forceps, which builds a fold of the bowel wall (Fig. 12.17). Using two graspers simultaneously, the tumor with the tumor-bearing wall is pulled inside the resection chamber. After localization of clear safety margins, the stapling function is activated, and with a knife, the semicircular resection is completed. The advantage of the FTRD device is that the bowel wall is already fused, and the vessels are occluded by the stapling mechanism before the wall is cut.

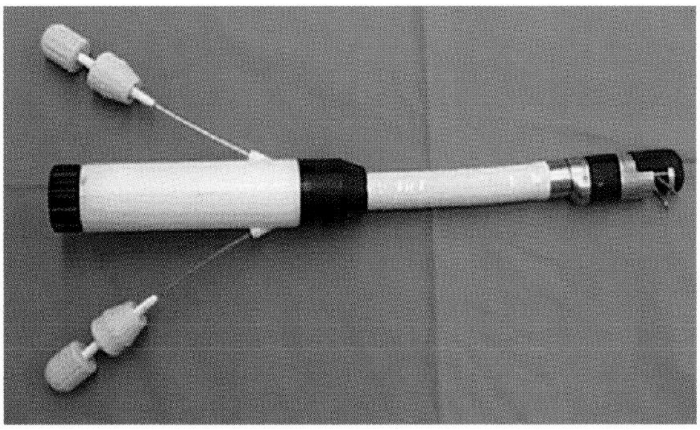

Fig. 12.16 The full-thickness resection device (FTRD). This instrument allows full -hickness stapling resection under endoscopic control

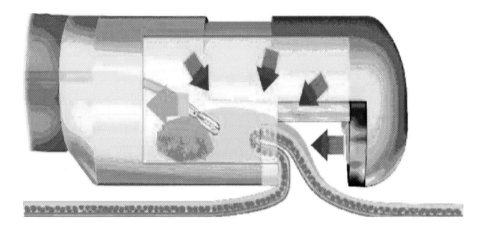

Fig. 12.17 Bowel wall in the resection chamber

This allows possible resection without any blood loss or risk of perirectal or pericolic infection. We have performed a series of animal experiments that allowed us to resect a bowel area of up to 6 cm in diameter, which means that tumors up to around 3 cm could be safely dissected with this device [20].

The development was stopped by Boston Scientific for different reasons. Our discussion dealt with the continuation of the program with the aim to make the stapling head thinner in diameter and more flexible, which would mean that the risk of moving upward into the descending colon would be reduced.

12.5   Conclusion

Endoscopic surgery has some systematic disadvantages, which have resulted in a relatively high complication rate in the starting phase of the application. Instruments that are more sophisticated and complex have been designed to compensate for the principle disadvantages of endoscopic surgery. The result of these new instruments is that endoscopic surgery can be performed much more precisely and much safer today.

It is, for example, clear today that the blood loss in endoscopic surgery is significantly less compared with open surgery because new hemostatic devices have been designed that permit dissection with minimum blood loss. Some years ago, companies started to design new devices for hemostatic dissection, based on the experience of endoscopic and open surgery.

The integration of more and more advanced technologies into combination instruments such as the FTRD device will in the future also allow the performing of procedures on an outpatient basis instead of highly complex laparoscopic colonic resections, which still have clear risks in the area of wound-healing problems at the anastomosis.

References

1. Breedveld P, Stassen HG, Meijer DW, Stassen LPS (1999) Theoretical background and conceptual solution for depth perception and eye–hand coordination problems in laparoscopic surgery. Min Invas Ther Allied Technol 8:227–234
2. Grimbergen CA, Jaspers JEN, Herder JL, Stassen HG (2001) Development of laparoscopic instruments. Min Invas Ther Allied Technol 10:145–154
3. Buess G, Kipfmuller K, Hack D, Grussner R, Heintz A, Junginger T (1988) Technique of transanal endoscopic microsurgery. Surg Endosc 2:71–75
4. Buess G, Kayser J (1995) Endoscopic Approach. Semin Laparosc Surg 2:268–274
5. Richard Wolf GmbH, Knittlingen, Germany. http://www.richard-wolf.com
6. Yokoyama M, Mailaender L, Raestrup H, Buess G (2003) Training system for laparoscopic fundoplication. Min Invas Ther Allied Technol 12:143–150
7. Schurr MO, Buess G, Schwarz K (2001) Robotics in endoscopic surgery: can mechanical manipulators provide a more simple solution for the problem of limited degrees of freedom? Min Invas Ther Allied Technol 10:289–293
8. Buess GF, Schurr MO, Fischer SC (2000) Robotics and allied technologies in endoscopic surgery. Arch Surg 135:229–235
9. Tübingen Scientific Medical GmbH, Tübingen, Germany. www.tuebingen-scientific.de
10. Inaki N (2004) Evaluation of a manual manipulator for endoscopic surgery – Radius Surgical System. Min Invas Ther Allied Technol 13:383
11. Waseda M (2004) Endoscopic suturing with a manual manipulator – Radius Surgical System. Min Invas Ther Allied Technol 13:384
12. Tuttlingen, Germany. www.aesculap.de
13. Arezzo A, Schurr MO, Braun A, Buess GF (2005) Experimental assessment of a new mechanical endoscopic solo-surgery system: Endofreeze. Surg Endosc 19:581–588
14. Buess G, Theiss R, Hutterer F, Pichlmaier H, Pelz C, Holfeld T, Said S, Isselhard W (1983) Transanal endoscopic surgery of the rectum – testing a new method in animal experiments. Leber Magen Darm 13:73–77
15. Buess GF, Raestrup H (2001) Transanal endoscopic microsurgery. Surg Oncol Clin N Am 10:709–731
16. ERBE Elektromedizin GmbH, Tübingen, Germany. www.erbe-med.de
17. Kanehira E, Raestrup H, Schurr MO, Wehrmann M, Manncke K, Buess GF (1993) Transanal endoscopic microsurgery using a newly designed multifunctional bipolar cutting and monopolar coagulating instrument. Endosc Surg Allied Technol 1:102–106
18. Schurr MO, Buess G, Raestrup H, Arezzo A, Buerkert A, Schell C, Adams R, Banik M (2001) Full thickness resection device (FTRD) for endoluminal removal of large bowel tumours: development of the instrument and related experimental studies. Min Invas Ther Allied Technol 10: 301–309
19. Boston Scientific Corporation, Natick, Mass. www.boston-scientific.com
20. Rajan E, Gostout CJ, Burgart LJ, Leontovich ON, Knipschiel MA, Herman LJ, Norton ID (2002) First endoluminal system for transmural resection of colorectal tissue with a prototype full-thickness resection device in a porcine model. Gastrointest Endosc 55:915–920

New Hemostatic Dissecting Forceps with a Metal Membrane Heating Element

13

Eiji Kanehira and Toru Nagase

13.1 Introduction

Quick and safe division of vessels is mandatory for advanced endoscopic surgery. Ultrasonically activated devices (USADs) [1–3] or bipolar vessel sealers (BVSs) [4–6] have been proven useful devices for hemostatic dissection in advanced endoscopic operations. But there are still some drawbacks associated with these dissecting devices. To overcome these drawbacks, we have been developing a new surgical device that does not utilize ultrasonic vibration or high frequency. What facilitates vessel sealing in our new device is the heat produced in a metal membrane. In this chapter, a prototype of the new device we have been working on for endoscopic operations is introduced, and its ability and performance in hemostatic dissection assessed in animal experiments is demonstrated.

13.2 Materials and Methods

The system developed for the laboratory use includes the recent prototype of dissecting forceps designed for endoscopic operation, a power controller, a connecting cable, and a foot switch (Fig. 13.1)

The prototype forceps used for the current test are designed like the Maryland dissecting forceps commonly used in endoscopic operations (Fig. 13.2a). Its shaft is 5 mm in maximum diameter, to be inserted through a 5-mm port. However, a 10-mm port had to be used instead of a 5-mm one in the current experiment because the lead wires for the electricity have not been installed inside the shaft. The forceps are composed of a pair of grippers at the tip, a shaft, and a pair of ring handles to open and close the grippers. The grippers, made of stainless steel, are curved to facilitate

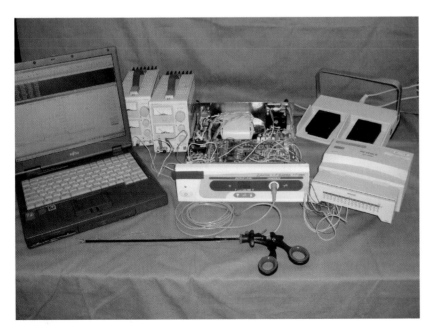

Fig. 13.1 The prototype hemostatic system used for the current experiments includes dissecting forceps for endoscopic operations, a power controller, a connecting cable, and a foot switch

tissue dissection, mimicking those of the Maryland dissecting forceps. One of the grippers is equipped with a metal blade with a relatively dull edge (Fig. 13.2b). A small heating resistor element is built into the blade. This element, a thin metal membrane, is made of molybdenum. Lead wires connect the heating element to the connecting cable. When electric energy is given to the molybdenum membrane, it produces heat, heating the blade. It is the most unique point of our new device, that the blade produces heat, no matter whether the blade contacts the tissue or not. In contrast, other commonly used devices, such as monopolar high-frequency devices, bipolar vessel sealers, or ultrasonically activated devices, need to contact tissue to generate Joule heat or frictional heat. The surface of the blade is coated with fluoroplastic to prevent char sticking. The opposed gripper is equipped with a tissue pad made of elastic silicone to receive the blade (Fig. 13.2c). When a vessel is clamped between the blade and the tissue pad and the blade is heated, the vessel is closed, welded, and sealed. Then the elasticity of the silicone pad allows the blade to cut into the vessel, and finally, the vessel is divided.

The power controller regulates the electric power to let the heating element emit the desired heat. The time-versus-temperature curve, we presume ideal for hemostatic tissue dissection, is like the one obtained by ultrasonically activated device. So we set the program of the power controller in order to obtain such time-versus-temperature curve in the tissue, which gradually goes up and exceeds the water boiling point in about several seconds, reaching around 200°C in about 10 s. To obtain such time versus-temperature-curve, the temperature difference between the heating element and the contacting tissue has to be considered. Considering this temperature gradient, we set the maximum temperature of the heating membrane higher than 300°C.

A female pig weighing 61 kg was given general anesthesia and used for the current experiments. The first experiment was performed to assess the device's performance for tissue dissection in the laparoscopic operation. For this task several portions of the mesenterium, omentum, and the root of the inferior mesenteric vessels were dissected, sealed, and divided. The next experiment was for assessing the ability and security in sealing the small- to medium-sized vessels. This task was performed under laparotomy, and the gastroepiploic arteries measuring 3 to 4 mm in outer diameter were sealed and divided by the new dissecting forceps. Output voltage, current, and time required to seal and cut each artery were measured and recorded. The maximum temperature that the heating element was supposed to reach was theoretically calculated in each session. For the sealing security experiment we harvested each artery segment cut by the heating forceps. The harvested arteries were immediately submitted to the following process. A cannula was inserted into the artery segment through the end opposite the occluded stump. The cannulation site was closed tightly with

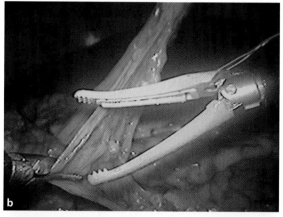

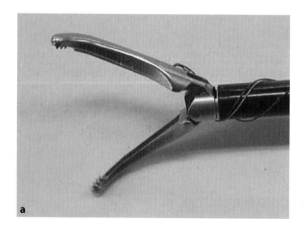

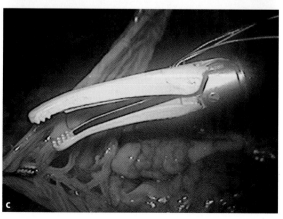

Fig. 13.2 a Closeup of the prototype forceps. The grippers are ideally curved as in the conventional dissecting forceps. **b** In one of the grippers a heating blade is attached. In the blade a heating element, made of molybdenum, is built in. **c** Closeup of the prototype forceps. In the opposed gripper an elastic tissue pad (*black part*) is equipped to receive the blade

clamping forceps. The cannula was connected both to a syringe and a digital manometer. The artery segment, digital manometer, syringe, and the connection tubes were filled with normal saline and sealed off to become a closed system. By slowly pushing the piston of the syringe, the artery's intraluminal pressure was increased until the occluded vessel burst. The time versus-pressure-curve was demonstrated on the computer monitor and recorded. The peak of the time–pressure curve was defined as the burst pressure of the artery segment.

In addition, we examined the artery stump by microscope. The artery was fixed in paraffin and stained with hematoxylin and eosin.

13.3   Results

Dissection and hemostatic division of the mesenterium and omentum in the laparoscopic setting was excellently performed by the new dissecting forceps. The

curved grippers seemed significantly advantageous in dissecting around the target tissue. Although a small amount of smoke was detected when the device was activated and the target was treated, it did not obscure the endoscopic view as much as the mist produced by the USAD. We touched the living tissue such as the intestinal wall or liver with the tip of the device while it was activated. Because no cavitation phenomenon is associated with our device, we did not see such injury in the tissue, which the device tip contacted, as seen in the tissue destroyed by the USAD's cavitation. The only change we saw in the surface of the touched tissue was that the point was discolored whitish.

The root of the inferior mesenteric artery, measuring approximately 7 mm in diameter, was sealed and cut by the new device. It was well demonstrated that this large-sized artery could be securely sealed and divided in one session (Fig. 13.3a–d).

In the latter experiment, 12 portions of the medium-sized arteries (gastroepiploic arteries), measuring 3 to 4 mm in diameter, were sealed and cut by the proto-

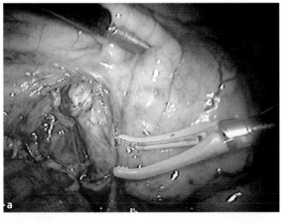
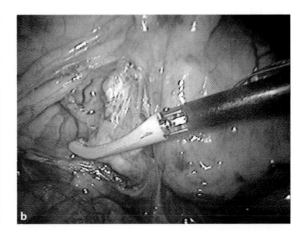
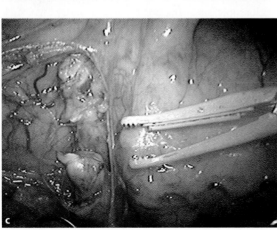
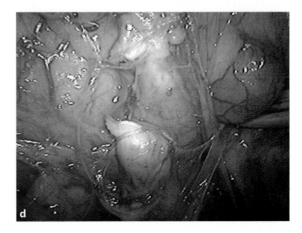

Fig. 13.3 a The root of the porcine inferior mesenteric artery (IMA), measuring approximately 7 mm in outer diameter. The curved forceps facilitated fine dissection. **b** The porcine IMA was clamped by the forceps, and ideal heat for sealing was be-

ing given to the IMA. **c** The IMA could be sealed and divided. **d** Closeup of the cut edge of the porcine IMA. The stump was sufficiently sealed, tolerating the arterial pressure

Time and bursting pressure

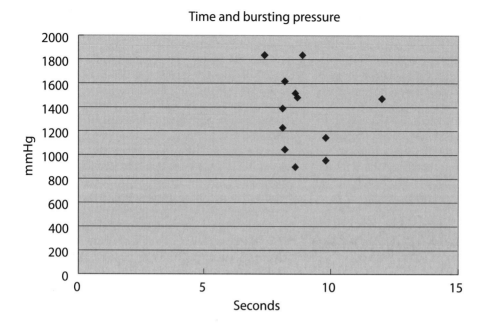

Fig. 13.4 Distribution of burst pressures in 12 artery segments and time required to seal and cut each artery

type forceps. All portions were sufficiently sealed and cut without hemorrhage.

Time required sealing and cutting the artery ranged from 8.2 to 12 s, with an average of 8.9 s (Fig. 13.4).

In the manometry experiments two stumps were not burst by the maximum pressure of the manometer system (1,839 mmHg). The other 10 stumps showed burst pressures ranging from 897 to 1,618 mmHg (Fig. 13.4).

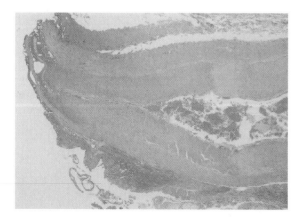

Fig. 13.5 Microscopic picture of the porcine artery sealed and divided by the prototype forceps (high-power view, hematoxylin and eosin staining). The artery was well welded, closed, and cut without carbonization, vacuolization, or severe desiccation

Microscopic examination revealed that the artery stump was sufficiently denatured, welded, and closed (Fig. 13.5). The tissue denature was not associated with such extreme changes such as carbonization, vacuolization, or severe desiccation, often characteristically observed in monopolar high-frequency technique.

13.4   Discussion

Endoscopic surgeons are becoming aware that such new hemostatic dissecting devices as USADs or BVSs are the key devices for advanced endoscopic operations, which require coagulation and division of many vessels [1–6]. When all vessels have to be ligated and divided by knot tying or clipping, the procedure becomes significantly time-consuming and requires much expertise.

Although these new hemostatic dissecting devices have been widely welcomed by surgeons, there are some drawbacks. As far as USADs are concerned, the risk of the cavitation phenomenon occurring at the tip of the vibrating blade, must be cautioned [7]. This ultrasonic vibration–specific phenomenon has as tissue destructive effect and may result in adjacent organ injury. Besides, ultrasonic vibration generates mist. The ultrasonic vibration breaks the links among water molecules in the tissue and eventually causes the mist. The mist obscures the operation field during endoscopic surgery. Moreover, the mist has potential hazard to transmit infectious material to the atmosphere [8] and to possibly disseminate viable cells [9].

In BVSs designed for endoscopic operations, two actions are needed to achieve coagulation and cutting. After coagulating the vessel one has to slide the cutter to cut the target. Moreover when the cutting function is integrated, the gripper must be straight because a cutter has to slide straight along the gripper. And when the gripper is curved for facilitating tissue dissection, cutting function has to be abandoned. The similar drawback is also pointed out in USADs. The active blade of a USAD must be straight or almost straight to transmit the ultrasonic vibration effectively. Freedom for the shape of the end effecter in these devices is limited.

Reflecting on all those drawbacks associated with the conventional hemostatic dissecting forceps, our main aims in the current development of a new hemostatic dissecting forceps are set: (1) not to have cavitation phenomenon, (2) not to produce mist, and (3) to have freedom in shape. In order to achieve all these goals, we decided not to use ultrasonic vibration or high-frequency electrocautery as its energy source.

The reason why we started to test the metal membrane heating element as an alternative energy is that we thought it would be possible to control the heat by giving the controlled power to this element and to obtain the similar time-versus-temperature curve as in the USAD technique. We have reported that the heat produced by a USAD is considerably milder, and it increases the temperature more gradually than does the heat produced by conventional monopolar electrocautery [10]. It was reported that the heat produced by a BVS is also significantly milder than is the conventional monopolar high-frequency technique [11]. As extremely rapid increase in temperature results in boiling the water in the cells, their subsequent explosion and eventually desiccation of tissue, it is not ideal for tissue welding [12]. On the other hand, when the temperatures lower than the boiling point are reached, protein and intracellular water denature into glue-like material.

Our development group has already investigated in previous experiments and reported that the metal membrane heating element made of molybdenum can emit adequate temperatures to seal vessels sufficiently [13]. The basic concept and principle for the current study have not been changed from the previous ones. We brought the same technology into the shape compatible for endoscopic surgery, making necessary parts thinner. As a heating element, molybdenum membrane is again used. The main change in the power controller was to set the program for emitting constant voltage, while in the previous experiments it was driven to obtain the constant temperature. This change

was introduced mainly because we found that in the constant temperature setting, the energy given to the tissue is decreased in the latter half of the activating period, when more energy should be needed for cutting the target. Interestingly in the constant voltage setting, we found the time-versus-temperature curve is more similar to those in USAD technique, and energy given to the tissue for the latter half of the activating period is higher.

When compared with previous reports on the ability of a USAD to seal the vessel, the ability of our new device seems equivalent or even higher [14–16]. The minimal burst pressure recorded in our experiment was 897 mmHg, which is much higher than the normal blood pressure of a living animal. In addition, the time required to seal and cut the vessels by our new device was as short as by the USAD technique. Interestingly, the microscopic findings in the artery stump obtained in the current experiments were remarkably similar to those obtained by a USAD in our previous experiments [14].

Advantages of our new device, compared with USADs, were clearly seen in the current experiments. It does produce a little amount of smoke, although it does not significantly disturb the operation, whereas the mist produced by USAD disturbs the procedure frequently. The fact that the cavitation phenomenon is never seen in our new device should make the dissection procedure significantly safer than the USAD procedure.

Like BVSs, the shape of the end effecter in our device can be made as curved as surgeons wish for their utility. And in our device this utility with the curved shape does not have to be compromised by the cutting function. Another advantage of our device is that both functions, sealing and cutting, are achieved in one action, while this utility is not integrated in BVSs. When also compared with the high-frequency techniques, there are advantages seen in our device. From the viewpoint of "electrical security", our device, which emits no electric current, should be safer than the current electrocautery, in which high-frequency electric current is transmitted in the human body, although it occurs only between the two electrodes in the bipolar technique. During tissue dissection near the nerve system, for example, our device is considered to be advantageous. Another unique advantage of our device is that the surface of the blade can be coated with fluoroplastic to prevent char sticking. The end effecter of the other electric devices cannot be coated because the electric current has to be discharged through the surface of the end effecter.

We are bringing this development to the next stage in order to assess the stability, durability, and feasibility as a commercial good. And the development is also focused on establishing the same system for open surgery. The endoscopic version as well as the open version is expected to pass further subjects or tests, and to be put into clinical trial in near future.

Acknowledgment

The authors are grateful to all staffs of Therapeutic Products Development Department, Research & Development Division, Olympus Medical Systems Corporation, Tokyo, Japan, for their enthusiastic support of the current experiments.

References

1. Amaral JF (1993) Laparoscopic application of an ultrasonically activated scalpel. Gastrointest Clin No Am 3:381–392
2. Kanehira E, Omura K, Kinoshita T, Sasaki M, Watanabe T, Kawakami K, Watanabe Y (1998) Development of a 23.5-kHz ultrasonically activated device for laparoscopic surgery. Min Invas Ther Allied Technol 7:315–319
3. Gossot, D, Buess G, Cuschieri A, Leporte E, Lirici M, Marvic R, Meijer D, Melzer A, Scurr MO (2000) Ultrasonic dissection for endoscopic surgery. EAES Technology Group. Surg Endosc 14:968–969
4. Kennedy JS, Stranahan PL, Taylor KD, Chandler JG (1998) High-burst-strength, feedback-controlled bipolar vessel sealing. Surg Endosc 12:876–878
5. Remorgida V, Anserini P, Prigione S et al (1999) The behaviour of plastic-insulated instruments in electrosurgery: an overview. Min Invas Ther Allied Technol 8:77–81
6. Romano F, Caprotti R, Franciosi C, De Fina S, Colombo G, Uggeri F (2002) Laparoscopic splenectomy using Ligasure. Preliminary experience. Surg Endosc 16:1608–1611
7. Kanehira E, Kinishita T, Omura K (2000) Fundamental principles and pitfalls linked to the use of ultrasonic scissors. Ann Chir 125:363–369
8. Ott DE, Moss E, Martinez K (1998) Aerosol exposure from an ultrasonically activated (Harmonic) device. J Am Assoc Gynecol Laparosc 5:29–32
9. Nduka CC, Poland N, Kennedy M et al (1998) Does the ultrasonically activated scalpel release viable airborne cancer cells? Surg Endosc 12:1031–1034
10. Kinoshita T, Kanehira E, Omura K, Kawakami K, Watanabe Y (1999) Experimental study on heat production by a 23.5-kHz ultrasonically activated device for endoscopic surgery. Surg Endosc 13:621–625
11. Campbell PA, Cresswell AB, Frank TG, Cuschieri A (2003) Real-time thermography during energized vessel sealing and dissection. Surg Endosc 17:1640–1645
12. Sigel B, Dunn MR The mechanism of blood vessel closure by high frequency electrocoagulation. Surg Gynecol Obstet 121:823–831
13. Kanehira E, Kinoshita T, Inaki N, Sekino N, Iida K, Omura K (2002) Development of a new hemostatic dissecting forceps utilizing controlled heat as an energy source. Min Invas Ther Allied Technol 11:243–247
14. Kanehira E, Omura K, Kinoshita T, Kawakami K, Watanabe Y (1999) How secure are the arteries occluded and divided by a newly designed ultrasonically activated device. Surg Endosc 13:340–342
15. Spivak H, Richardson WS, Hunter JG (1998) The use of bipolar cautery, laparosonic coagulating shears, and vascular clips for hemostasis of small and medium sized vessels. Surg Endosc 12:183–185
16. Harold KL, Pollinger H, Matthews BD, Kercher KW, Sing RF, Heniford BT (2003) Comparison of ultrasonic energy, bipolar thermal energy, and vascular clips for hemostasis of small-, medium-, and large-sized arteries. Surg Endosc 17:1228–1230

Radiofrequency and Hepatic Tumors

14

Piero Rossi and Adriano De Majo

14.1 Introduction

Follow-up and monitoring program and progress in imaging have made notable contributions to early and accurate diagnosis of primitive and metastatic neoplastic nodules of the liver. Today, the indications for surgical resection of patients suffering from hepatocarcinoma and metastases (colorectal and non-colorectal) are well codified.

The refinement of image-based diagnostic methods and thin-needle biopsy techniques have permitted the development of guided therapeutic systems, in which the therapeutic agent is introduced directly into the lesion (interstitial therapies), with the aim of destroying the neoplastic tissue, leaving the healthy surrounding parenchyma. Cellular death can be caused by cytotoxic damage (ethanol, acetic acid) or by heat damage (laser, cryotherapy, microwaves, radiofrequency). Percutaneous ethanol injection has acquired proven efficacy in the treatment of HCC [1].

Thermoablation by means of radiofrequencies (RFA), described initially for the treatment of small intracranial lesions, osteoid osteomas, rhizotomies, and cordotomies, was successively experimented on animal and then human liver in the treatment of small HCC [2]. It consists of the destruction of the neoplastic tissue by means of the action of heat generated by an active needle electrode introduced into the neoplastic tissue itself, high-frequency alternating current flowing from an electrode into the surrounding tissue. Frictional heating is caused when the ions in the tissue attempt to follow the changing directions of the alternating current. In the mononopolar mode, current flows from the electrode to a round pad applied externally to the skin. In the bipolar mode, current passes between two electrodes inserted at opposite poles of the tumor.

The needle electrode can be positioned percutaneously (under ultrasound or TC guidance), by laparoscopy or open laparotomy. It is connected to an appropriate generator and is insulated, except for the terminal part (active). The active electrode has a thermocouple on the point to constantly monitor the temperature. The energy emitted inside the tissue is converted into heat that causes cell death by means of coagulative necrosis. At 43°C in 30–60 s apoptosis already is seen. Cellular death occurs in a few minutes at 50°C; in a few seconds at 55°C, and almost instantaneously at temperatures above 60°C.

The destruction of a limited volume of tissue is thus realizable in a controlled and reproducible manner. Heating of the tissue decreases in proportion to the fourth power of the distance from the electrodes. Charring causes sudden rise in impedance adjacent to the electrode.

Many strategies exist for increasing the size of ablation volume (enlarge the zone of ablation):
- Cooling the electrode to avoid charring and increase of impedance
- Cluster cooled electrode
- Expandable jack hook needles

There are various types of electrodes commercially available: cooled tip, single and triple (cluster) and expandable needles [3–5].

The diameter of the volume of necrosis must be greater than that of the neoplastic nodule by at least 5–10 mm. Imaging techniques are important to localize the tumor and to monitor the ablation process. Typically, the electrode is placed under ultrasound or CT.

During ablation, ultrasound monitoring shows a round hyperechoic area.

This phenomenon depends, according to some writers, on the vaporization of the interstitial liquid and to others on the out-gassing of dissolved nitrogen in the tissue that is roughly proportionate to the volume of necrosis (Fig. 14.1).

To verify destruction of the tumor after RFA we recommend high-resolution, good-quality contrast enhanced CT or MR to evaluate completeness and recurrence rates [6] (Fig. 14.2).

Published studies are principally directed at criteria of feasibility, efficacy, safety, and survival (even if the follow-ups are still short) [6–8].

RFA is currently directed at those patients for whom resection is not suitable. As part of a mandatory multidisciplinary approach, RFA must be seen within the

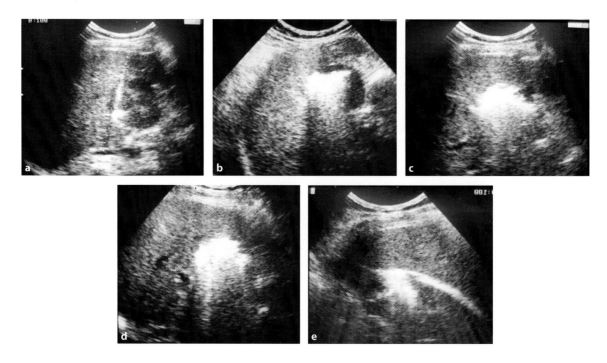

Fig. 14.1 RFA of HCC. US monitoring: hyperechoic area that gradually covers the entire nodule (**a–d**). Bubbles eventually run in hepatic vein (**e**)

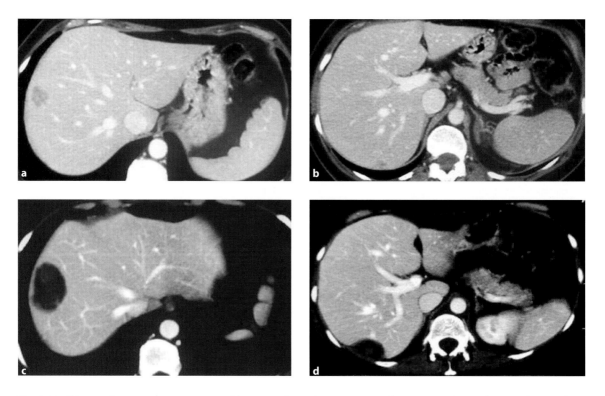

Fig. 14.2 CT pre and posttreatment in 55-year-old patient subjected to anterior rectal resection and RFA of two synchronous liver metastases (**a, b**). Complete necrosis occurred (**c, d**)

therapeutic algorithm of primitive and metastatic tumors of the liver.

The advantages of RFA are the saving of healthy liver, the mini-invasiveness of the method itself, the repeatability, the limited costs, the feasibility also in patients for whom resection is not suitable with reduced morbidity, and almost nil mortality.

The laparoscopic approach has been proposed as an alternative to the percutaneous approach in selected patients; it permits better staging (24% lesions not diagnosed by TC) and a safer approach for lesions that are not safely treatable percutaneously (subcapsular, near the hollow viscera etc.) [9].

Analogously, the laparotomic approach permits better staging; access to segments I, VII, and VIII; the protection of surrounding viscera; vascular control maneuvers (Pringle); and, further, association with the resective surgery itself.

Orthotopic liver transplant (OLT) permits treatment of both hepatocarcinoma and cirrhosis. It is indicated in patients with early HCC (single nodule ≤5 cm, or <3 nodules ≤3 cm). However, because of the limited number of organs, average waiting time is over 1 year. Surgical resection therefore remains the fundamental therapeutic option.

Transarterial chemoembolization (TACE) is used for patients with hypervascularized multiple nodules. Alcoholization (percutaneous ethanol injection [PEI]) is indicated in nodules of small dimensions.

RFA initially used as an alternative to PEI [1, 10, 11] has rapidly gained ground and is currently included in the HCC therapeutic algorithm both as curative therapy (European Consensus Conference, Barcelona) and as a bridge to OLT [12–14].

Histological investigations on removed livers have validated RFA as an efficacious treatment in small HCCs (≤3 cm) [15]. Further, interstitial therapies such as PEI or RFA can be integrated with TACE.

Hepatic metastases can be divided into colorectal and non-colorectal. Twenty to 30% of patients with colorectal carcinoma develop hepatic metastases; only 10–20% are respectable, and hepatic resection is the therapeutic gold standard [16–18].

Regarding those from non-colorectal tumors, indication for resective surgery is straightforward for testicular, renal, and neuroendocrine tumors (NET) [19].

Hepatectomy for metastases from other primitive tumors appears to be appropriate for metastases from some sarcomas, mammary carcinomas and the gynecological sphere, and lastly from melanoma, but the selection criteria are still little defined.

The criterion of nonresectability must be expressed by a surgeon expert in the field of hepatic surgery. For patients for whom resection is not available, ablative techniques can provide a therapeutic alternative.

Further, RFA has gained growing application in association with hepatic resection itself.

In general, in connection with colorectal carcinoma metastases, RFA can be indicated in patients not suitable for resection for general reasons; for anesthesiological reasons; for location, number, and vascular relationships of the lesions; for patient refusal; in association with resection of the primitive tumor; in association with hepatic resection of other nodules; and finally, in local recurrences following surgery.

Elias [20] reports his clinical experience with intraoperative RFA associated with hepatectomy to treat otherwise unresectable liver metastases with curative intent. The same author states [21] that well-used RFA is at least as efficient as wedge resections to treat liver metastases smaller than 3 cm.

At the same time, it is clear that RFA is better tolerated than is wedge resection, is less invasive, is less hemorrhagic, and does not necessitate vascular clamping. It could thus be currently considered a valid tool in the arsenal of intraoperative procedures to treat liver metastases. The combination of anatomical segmental and wedge resections, RFA, and optimal chemotherapy in patients with technically unresectable LM results in median survival of 36 months [22].

Analogically, Oshowo and Gillams report that RFA used in conjunction with surgery, in patients who were regarded as "nonsurgical" due to the extent and distribution of their disease, gives results similar to those reported for patients undergoing resection for operable liver metastases. They concluded that RFA extend the scope of surgical treatment in patients previously thought to be unsuitable for surgical resection [23].

Tepel [24], in 26 patients with 88 hepatic lesions, concluded that intraoperative RFA alone, or in combination with liver resection, extends the spectrum of liver surgery in cases where complete resection is not possible.

Our case experience consists of 37 patients with 65 HCC nodules, 5 patients affected with cholangiocarcinoma, and 63 patients with 115 metastatic lesions originating from various primitive tumors (40 patients with colorectal carcinoma; 10 patients with breast carcinoma; 6 patients with gastric neoplasia, 4 of which with carcinoma, 1 with gastrointestinal stromal tumor [GIST] and 1 with NET; 2 patients with renal carcinoma; 2 with oesophageal carcinoma; 2 with pancreatic cancer; and 1 with anal cancer.

Regarding HCC, there were 55 procedures, of which 52 were carried out percutaneously, 2 by laparotomy, and 1 by laparoscopic approach.

In the field of metastatic lesions, there were 85 procedures, of which 58 were percutaneous and 27 laparotomic.

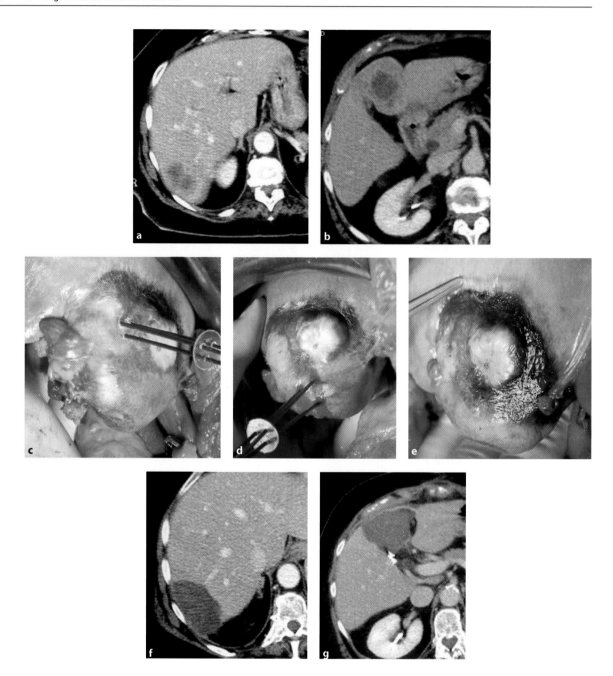

Fig. 14.3 A 71-year-old patient, subjected to left colectomy and RFA of two synchronous metastases. **a, b** CT preoperative scan. **c–e** Intraoperative RFA by cluster; **e** shows the hyperechoic ring around necrotic area. **f, g** CT scan shows complete necrosis

All the procedures were performed with a Radionics generator and cooled-tip electrodes, single or cluster (triple).

Complete necrosis, evaluated through TC with vascular contrast medium, analogically to the data in the literature, was obtained in almost all of the nodules ≤3 cm.

In addition, with a view to evaluating the feasibility of RFA in synchronous metastases from colorectal carcinoma, 10 patients with 36 nodules (range: 1–10) were treated.

Intestinal resection was always effected prior to ablation (Fig. 14.3).

The necrosis obtained was complete in all nodules except for one with diameter >6 cm.

In our experience, open RFA is effective and safe, the use of the cluster is facilitated, numerous nodules can be treated, vascular control maneuvers can be carried out, and it is easier to evaluate intraoperatively the completeness of the necrosis [25–29].

As stated earlier, given the present state of knowledge, RFA can be considered as a curative treatment of HCC. Its impact in terms of survival in connection with hepatic metastases remains to be determined.

Gillams [30] studied the impact on survival by image-guided thermal ablation, using interstitial laser photocoagulation in patients with metastases from colorectal metastases not suitable for surgical resection. This therapy improved survival both when compared with systemic and regional chemotherapy results.

Oshowo compared outcome in patients with solitary colorectal liver metastases treated by surgery or RFA [31]. The contraindications at surgery were lesion close to or involving a major vessel (nine patients, comorbidity [nine], and stable extrahepatic disease [seven]). Patients who had liver resection had truly solitary metastases with no evidence of extrahepatic disease. Preliminary survival curves between the two groups were similar.

Abdalla examined recurrence and survival rates in patient treated with hepatic resection only, RFA plus resection, or RFA only for colorectal liver metastases. He concluded that the RFA alone or in combination with resection for unresectable patients does not provide survival comparable to resection and is only slightly superior to nonsurgical treatment [32].

Positive results in terms of survival are given by Berber with respect to systemic chemotherapy alone [33].

Poston [34], however, posed crucial questions in this field:

- Is destructive therapy equal in curability to surgery for resectable colorectal liver metastases?
- What additional survival benefit does destructive therapy have over modern systemic chemotherapy (oxaliplatin and irinotecan) in the treatment of unresectable disease?

Trials to attempt to answer these questions are ongoing.

After the initial phase centered on the feasibility and efficacy of the method, important multicentric investigations were carried out, from which on the one hand precise data regarding complications and mortality emerged, and on the other opportune guidelines.

Mulier reports a mortality rate of 0.5%, with complications of 8.9% [35].

Livraghi reports a mortality rate of 0.25%, with major complications of 2.1% and minor of 4.7% [36].

Even if it is widely recognized that the mechanism of cell destruction induced by RFA is sustained by necrosis and apoptosis mechanisms, the effective biological processes that result from this are not clear. RFA induces an inflammatory response in the site of application, thus modulating the cellular components of the immune system. Moreover RFA application seems to enhance antitumor immunity. In collaboration with our colleagues of the University of Rome La Sapienza, we have shown that leukocyte subsets differently respond to RFA application; in particular CD3/CD4 cells and CD19+ cells decrease following RFA in metastatic liver patients, while no such modulation is observed in HCC patients. Moreover an antigen specific antitumor immune response mediated by interferon (IFN)-γ production can be augmented following RFA [37].

With a view to obtaining greater volumes of necrosis, compared with monopolar RFA, from January to June 2003 at the Department of Biology, Animal Facility Centre (STA) University of Rome Tor Vergata, we started a series of experimentations on ex vivo pig liver, adopting multiple needle electrodes in bipolar mode. The preliminary results obtained from this experimentation led us to realize that multiple electrode needles arranged comb fashion would realize slices of parenchymal coagulation with closure of the blood and biliary vessels in a reasonable time, avoiding multiple applications of a single monopolar needle.

In these procedures RF electrosurgical apparatus in bipolar mode was used to produce a sinusoidal pure wave of 660-kHz frequency, 140-V output, and maximum power of 30 W, with 100-Ω impedance that fed two electrodes.

The entire system was originally composed of three RF generators and six electrodes. Finally, we fashioned a single generator that was modified to deliver 60 W, through six electrodes with 500-Ω impedance, and forced cooling. The apparatus was modified in order to supply controlled power simultaneously to five bipolar circuits through the six electrodes that constituted the application tool, fed from an output transformer with six terminals. The following parameters were evaluated: distance between electrodes, energy delivered, width and thickness of necrosis, and needle diameter. After the approval of the Animal Ethics Committee, 18 liver resections on six pigs (Landrace pig) were performed from September 2003 to December 2004. All procedures were performed under general anesthesia, with tracheal intubation and continuous cardiac monitoring, with midline laparotomy and without vascular control. Nine atypical liver resections were performed in three animals sacrificed at the end of the experiments. Nine atypical liver resections were performed in three animals, at two different times. The animals were kept alive after primary operation to evaluate the principal complications (bleeding, biliary leakage). Blood sampling was performed before the first operation, and at the fourth postoperative day to assess bleeding.

During the second operation, we carefully evaluated the entire abdominal cavity and the liver edge, performing biopsy of the necrotic tissue (for histologi-

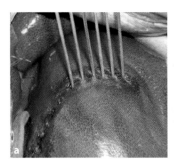
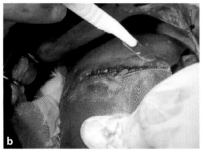
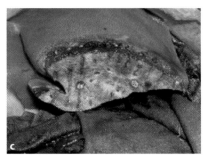

Fig. 14.4 a Single line coagulation in left lateral lobe in pig's liver. **b** Section with scalpel along the necrotic line. **c** Liver edge after resection

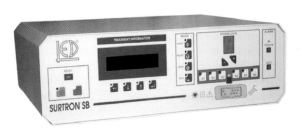
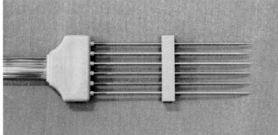

Fig. 14.5 Bipolar automatic generator and comb

cal control), and carried out another two resections on each animal.

The resections were performed with a normal scalpel after multiple application of the multielectrode probe along the established line (Fig. 14.4).

In order to obtain optimal coagulation of the slice of liver parenchyma, and to facilitate the cutting of the tissue, we decided to perform a double parallel line of application of the probe.

During this phase we used a generator with 475 kHz, 160 V, and 150 W (SURTRON SB) (Fig. 14.5).

Finally, to access the tolerability and safety of the system on human beings, after IRB approval, we designed and implemented a clinical pilot study in our institution. In connection with the feasibility, we looked at the coagulative panel and intra- and postoperative echo color Doppler blood flow results. With regard to the efficacy, we studied the extent of the coagulative necrosis, blood loss, and the healing of the transected liver as well as the handling of the probes.

We obtained the approval of the Hospital Ethical Committee and the informed consent of each patient. The preoperative work up was standard for surgery of hepatic tumors. Postoperative controls involved evaluation of the blood count, liver enzymes, and coagulation panels. Ultrasound examination allowed us to evaluate collection and hepatic vessel flow. Finally, the CT scan gave us evaluation of the liver edge (Fig. 14.6).

The study included the enrolment of six patients with primary and metastatic tumors suitable for liver resection according to the usual surgical criteria for these cases. Four patients had colorectal metastases, one patient suspected gallbladder carcinoma, and one patient suspected intrahepatic cholangiocarcinoma.

Altogether, the following procedures were carried out: three left lobectomies, one left hepatectomy, one gallbladder bed resection, and four wedge resections. Associated surgery was RFA in two unresectable tumors, one total colectomy, and one ileocoloanastomosis. Whenever possible, ligation, and division of the inflow vessels was performed before transection, allowing rapid coagulation of the liver plane.

In the case of the left hepatectomy, we proceeded prudently, as it was our first patient and so performed control of portal left pedicle and left hepatic vein; in contrast, in last left lobectomy we performed resection without vascular control.

No vascular control was needed for the wedge resection. In the other patients only portal inflow control was obtained.

After the double line of tissue coagulation, we cut the liver parenchyma with a normal scalpel. Successive application of the probe allows transection close to the hepatic vein. Blood loss is minimal. The probe can be used also in an anteroposterior direction.

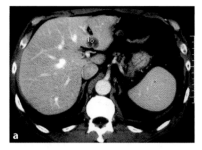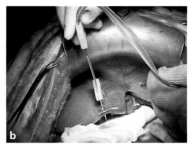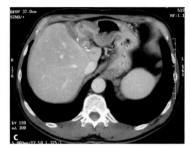

Fig. 14.6 A 68-year-old patient with metachronous metasta-ses from colonic cancer subjected to left hepatectomy. *Left to right* **a** Preoperative CT scan, **b** intraoperative coagulation of the liver resection plane, **c** postoperative CT scan after 1 month that shows necrotic tissue at liver edge

Close to the hepatic vein, coagulation is not prudent and so we transect the tissue in a traditional way.

The hepatic vein was divided by a stapler.

We observed only one complication in Patient 2, whose drainage was removed with output still at 100 ml. However, normalization came about after 45 days.

Recently, another three patients with colorectal liver metastases underwent liver resection using this device: two right hepatectomy and one right lateral segmentectomy plus RFA of nodule in the fourth segment.

In conclusion, the coagulation with multielectrode bipolar radiofrequency device allows a liver blood-less resection. Liver resection assisted by this device is feasible, easy, and safe. This method for liver resection is absolutely tolerable by the patient with no systemic complication or adverse reaction. This new technique offers a method for a blood less hepatic transection [38–42].

Currently, the generator is able to check the tissue impedance and thereby automatically choose the power. Further, still automatically, it can operate the switching out of each electrode as soon as necrosis is reached. The comb is relatively manageable; a special device has been realized in order to facilitate both the insertion and the protection of the hands of the surgeon, together with the surrounding organs. Thanks to the tissue necrosis, we can hypothesize a low level of recurrence at the level of the resected liver edge over the long term.

not suitable for surgical resection, and for low morbidity and mortality related to the ablation technique itself.

Information from experience and literature data gave us a lot of information in the field of tolerability, safety, efficacy, complications, and the possibility of specifying opportune guidelines.

Nevertheless many questions as to biological and therapeutic issues are still unsolved:

- Impact on long-term survival
- Relation to systemic inflammatory and immunologic response
- Imbrications with systemic or intra-arterial chemotherapy
- Immunotherapy
- Relation to other kind of interstitial therapy
- Relation to, or substitution of, surgical resection
- Benefits of debulking in conjunction with chemotherapy or other systemic therapy

RFA is actually the most versatile and most used form of interstitial therapy. It has found defined utilization in HCC treatments. Its role in the field of liver metastasis is still evolving, above all due to notable results with recent aggressive chemotherapy.

In the multidisciplinary approach to the solid liver tumor, RFA is a further important tool in the ongoing battle against cancer.

Definitive data should emerge from controlled clinical trials.

14.2   Conclusions

Oncological therapy of solid neoplasms is continuously evolving. Traditionally, local tumor removal has required major surgery. Recently, progress in imaging has permitted the development of interstitial therapies with "*in situ*" destruction of liver tumors and saving of normal tissue. In this scenario, RFA has received increasing interest, both for the possibilities of treating patients

References

1. Livraghi T, Golgberg SN, Lazzaroni S, Meloni F, Gazelle GS (1998) Small hepatocellular carcinoma: treatment with radio-frequency ablation versus ethanol injection. Radiology 210:655–661
2. Rossi S, Di Stasi M, Buscarini E, Quaretti P, Garbagnati F, Squassante L, Perercutaneous RF (1996) Interstitial thermal ablation in the treatment of hepatic cancer. Am J Roentgenol 167:759–768

3. Lencioni R, Cioni D, Bartolozzi C (2001) Percutaneous radiofrequency thermal ablation of liver malignancies: techniques, indications, imaging findings, and clinical results. Abdom Imaging 26:345–360

4. Nahum Goldberg S, Dupuy DE (2001) Image-guided radiofrequency tumor ablation: challenger and opportunities, part I. J Vasc Interv Radiol 12:1021–1032

5. Nahum Goldberg S, Dupuy DE (2001) Image-guided radiofrequency tumor ablation: challenger and opportunities, part II. J Vasc Interv Radiol 12:11351148

6. Catalano O, Lobianco R, Esposito M, Siani A (2001) Hepatocellular carcinoma recurrence after percutaneous ablation therapy: helical CT patterns. Abdom Imaging 26:375–383

7. Curley SA, Izzo F, Delrio P, Ellis LM, Granchi J, Vallone P, Fiore F, Pignata S, Daniele B, Cremona F (199) Radiofrequency ablation of unresectable primary and metastatic hepatic malignancies: results in 123 patients. Ann Surg 230:1–8

8. Curley SA, Izzo F, Vauthej JN, Vallone P (2000) Radiofrequency ablation of hepatocellular cancer in 110 patients with cirrhosis. Ann Surg 232:381–391

9. Santambrogio R, Padda M, Zuin M, Bertolini E, Bruno S, Cornalba GP, Costa M, Montorsi M (2003) Safety and efficacy of laparoscopic radiofrequency of hepatocellular carcinoma in patients with liver cirrhosis. Surg Endosc 17:1826–1832

10. Livraghi T, Goldberg SN, Lazzaroni S, Meloni F, Ierace T, Solbiati L, Gazelle GS (2000) Hepatocellular carcinoma: radio-frequency ablation of medium and large lesions. Radiology 214:761–768

11. Tateishi R, Shiina S, Teratani T, Obi S, Sato S, Koike Y, Fujishima T, Yoshida H, Kawabe T, Omata M (2005) Percutaneous radio-frequency ablation for hepatocellular carcinoma: an analysis of 1,000 cases. Cancer 103:1201–1209

12. Bruix J, Sherman M, Llovet JM, Beaugrand M, Lencioni R, Burroughs AK, Christensen E, Pagliaro L, Colombo M, Rodés J (2001) EASL Panel of Experts on HCC Clinical management of hepatocellular carcinoma. Conclusions of the Barcelona 2000 EASL conference. European Association for the Study of the Liver. J Hepatol 35:421–430

13. Llovet JM, Schwartz M, Mazzaferro V (2005) Resection and liver transplantation for hepatocellular carcinoma. Semin Liver Dis 25:181–200

14. Llovet JM (2004) Updated treatment approach to hepatocellular carcinoma. J Gastroenterol 40:225–235

15. DSK Lu, Yu NC, Raman SS, Limanond P, Lassman C, Murray K, Tong MJ, Amado RG, Busuttil RW (2005) Radiofrequency ablation of hepatocellular carcinoma: treatment success as defined by histologic examination of the explanted liver. Radiology 234:954–960

16. Malafosse R, Penna Ch, Cunha Sa, Nordlinger B (2001) Surgical management of hepatic metastases from colorectal malignancies. Ann Oncol 12:887–894

17. Penna Ch, Nordlinger B (2002) Surgery of liver metastases from colorectal cancer: new promises. Br Med Bull 64:127–140

18. Bentrem DJ, de Matteo RP, Blumgart LH (2005) Surgical therapy for metastatic disease to the liver. Annu Rev Med 56:139–156

19. Elias D, Cavalcanti de A, Eggenspieler P, Plaud B, Ducreux M, Spielman M, Theodore C, Bonvalot S, Lasser P (1998) Resection of liver metastases from a noncolorectal primary: indications and results based on 147 monocentric patients. J Am Coll Surg 187:487–493

20. Elias D, Goharin A, Otmany El, Taieb J, Duvillard P, Lasser P, de Baere T (2000) Usefulness of intraoperative radiofrequency thermoablation of liver tumours associated or not with hepatectomy. Eur J Surg Oncol 26:763–769

21. Elias D, Baton O, Sideris L, Matsuhisa T, Pocard M, Lasser P (2004) Local recurrences after intraoperative radiofrequency ablation of liver metastases: a comparative study with anatomic and wedge resections. Ann Surg Oncol 11:500–505

22. Elias D, Baton O, Sideris L, Boige V, Malka D, Liberale G, Pocard M, Lasser P (2005) Hepatectomy plus intraoperative radiofrequency ablation and chemotherapy to treat technically unresectable multiple colorectal liver metastases. J Surg Oncol 90:36–42

23. Oshowo A, Gillams AR, Lees WR, Taylor I (2003) Radiofrequency ablation extends the scope of surgery in colorectal liver metastases. EJSO 29:244–247

24. Tepel J, Hinz S, Klomp HJ, Kapischke M, Kremer B (2004) Intraoperative radiofrequency ablation (RFA) for irresectable liver malignancies. EJSO 30:551–555

25. Rossi P, Danza FM, Stolfi VM, Di Lorenzo N, Coscarella G, Manzelli A, Arturi A, De Lisa F, Prisco AL, Bock E, Gaspari AL (2001) Radiofrequency interstitial thermal ablation of metastatic liver tumours. CARS 2001 Computer Assisted Radiology and Surgery 15th International Congress and Exhibition ICC, Berlin, Germany, 27–30 June 2001

26. Rossi P, Manzelli A, Susanna F, Gaspari AL (2001) Trattameno termoablativo con radiofrequenza delle metastasi epatiche da tumori neuroendocrini [in Italian]. Atti del XXI Congresso Nazionale SIEC Palermo, 13–15 September 2001

27. Gaspari AL, Rossi P, Danza FM (2002) Il trattamento delle metastasi epatiche con radiofrequenza, I supplementi di Tumori, vol. 1, no. 3; May–June 2002 [in Italian]. 26th Congresso Nazionale SICO L'Aquila, 20–22 June 2002

28. Rossi P, Coscarella G, De Majo A, Marino V, Bock E, Gaspari A, Danza FM (2002) Trattamento dell'epatocarcinoma su cirrosi mediante radiofrequenza [in Italian]. Convegno Nazionale SIPAD (Società Italiana Patologia Apparato Digerente), Rome, 5–6 December 2002

29. Rossi P, Coscarella G, De Majo A, Stolfi VM, De Lisa F, Ercoli L, Gaspari AL (2004) Efficacia della radiofrequenza intraoperatoria nel trattamento delle metastasi epatiche sincrone da carcinoma colorettale, I supplementi di Tumori, vol. 3, no. 5: S59–S61, September–October 2004 [in Italian]. XXVIII Congresso Nazionale SICO; le nuove tecnologie in chirurgia oncologica, Trieste, 9–11 September 2004

30. Gillams AR, Lees WR (2000) Survival after percutaneous, image-guided, thermal ablation of hepatic metastases from colorectal cancer. Dis Colon Rectum 43:5

31. Oshowo A, Gillams AR, Harrison E, Lees WR, Taylor I (2003) Comparison of resection and radiofrequency ablation for treatment of solitary colorectal liver metastases. Br J Surg 90:1240–1243

32. Abdalla EK, Vauthey JN, Ellis LM, Ellis V, Pollock R, Broglio KR, Hesse K, Curley SA (2004) Recurrence and outcomes following hepatic resection, radiofrequency ablation, and combined resection/ablation for colorectal liver metastases. Ann Surg 396:818–27

33. Berber E, Pelley R, Siperstein AE (2005) Predictors of survival after radiofrequency thermal ablation of colorectal cancer metastases to the liver: a prospective study. J Clin Oncol 23:1358-1364

34. Poston GJ (2005) Radiofrequency ablation of colorectal liver metastases: where we really going? J Clin Oncol 23:1342–1344

35. Mulier S, Mulier P, Ni Y, Miao Y, Dupas B, Marchal G, De Wever I, Michel L (2002) Complication of radiofrequency coagulation of liver tumors. Br J Surg 89:1206–1222

36. Livraghi T, Solbiati L, Meloni MF, Gazelle GS, Halpern EF, Goldberg SN (2003) Treatment of focal liver tumors with percutaneous radio-frequency ablation: complications encountered in a multicenter study. Radiology 226:441–451

37. Rughetti A, Rahimi H, Rossi P, Frati L, Nuti M, Gaspari A, Danza FM, Ercoli L (2003) Modulation of blood circulating immune cells by radiofrequency tumor ablation. J Exp Clin Cancer Res 22(Suppl):247–250

38. Rossi P, De Majo A, Mattei M, Gaspari AL (2004) La resezione epatica mediante radiofrequenza bipolare: studi sperimentali su fegato di maiale, I supplementi di Tumori, vol. 3, no. 5: S56–S58, September–October 2004 [in Italian]. XXVIII Congresso Nazionale SICO; le nuove tecnologie in chirurgia oncologica, Trieste, 9–11 September 2004

39. Rossi P, Coscarella G, De Majo A, Stolfi VM, De Lisa F, Ercoli L, Gaspari AL (2004) Efficacia della radiofrequenza intraoperatoria nel trattamento delle metastasi epatiche sincrone da carcinoma colorettale, I supplementi di Tumori, vol. 3, no. 5: S59–S61, September–October 2004 [in Italian]. XXVIII Congresso Nazionale SICO; le nuove tecnologie in chirurgia oncologica, Trieste, 9–11 September 2004

40. Rossi P, De Majo A, Coscarella G, Manzelli A, Gaspari AL (2005) Reseccion epatica sin sangrado con dispositivo bipolar multielectrodo de radiofrequencia [in Italian]. 76th Congreso Argentino de Cirugia, Buenos Aires, 20–23 November 2005

41. Rossi P, De Majo A, Manzelli A, Coscarella G, Sica GS, Gaspari AL (2006) Bloodless hepatic resection with multielectrode bipolar radiofrequency device. World Conference on Interventional Oncology, Cernobbio-Como, 12–16 June 2006

42. Rossi P, De Majo A, Mauti A, Mauti P, Quattrini V, Mattei M, Tognoni V, Cenci L, Manzelli A, Di Lorenzo N, Gaspari AL (2006) Bloodless hepatic resection with automatic bipolar radiofrequency generation and multielectrode in line device. Minim Invasive Ther Allied Technol 2007; 16:1; 66–72

Technological Innovations in Kidney and Liver Living-Donor–Related Transplantation

15

Enrico Benedetti

15.1 Introduction

Recently, the field of organ transplantation has reached a high level of clinical success because of significant improvements in immunosuppressive strategies. However, in the last decade, no significant technical innovations have significantly modified the approach to clinical organ transplantation in the recipient's operation. The success of transplantation has widened the gap between potential candidates and available cadaver donor organs. In fact, since 1995 the number of cadaveric donors for kidney transplants in the United States reached a plateau at approximately 8,000 a year, while the number of potential recipients continues to grow exponentially. In liver transplantation, the trend is similar. Interestingly, the mortality rate on the waiting list was 14.7% in 1995, almost unchanged compared to 17.6 % in 2003. Clearly, the main obstacle to further expansion of organ transplantation is the lack of adequate number of cadaveric donors. The most successful strategy to mitigate the donor shortage has been a more extensive use of living donors. In fact, the recent growth in the number of kidney transplantations performed in the United States has been entirely supported by an increased number of living-donor–related transplants in the face of a static supply of cadaveric donors. According to a recent United Network for Organ Sharing (UNOS) report, the number of kidney transplants from living donors has increased from 2,851 in 1993 to 6,464 in 2003 [1, 2]. Furthermore, in the last few years, living-donor liver transplantation, originally limited to pediatric recipients, has been successfully applied to adults. Living-donor liver transplantation has contributed to the reduction of donor organ shortage, and has allowed treatment for patients previously excluded from liver transplantation (i.e., those with large liver tumors) [3–5].

In our judgment, the most important, recent technical innovations in the field of organ transplantation have been the result of the increased focus on safe and reliable procurement of donor organs from living donors.

The aim of this chapter is to illustrate the impact of modern technologies in surgical techniques related to kidney and liver grafts procurement from living donors. In particular, it describes in detail laparoscopic robotic-assisted techniques for living-donor nephrectomy for kidney transplantation, as well as new strategies for safe parenchymal transection in hepatectomy for living donor liver transplantation.

15.2 Robotic Technology in Laparoscopic Living-Donor Nephrectomy

From its introduction in Boston in 1954 by Murray, living-donor nephrectomy performed in an open fashion has proven over the years to be a safe and effective procedure. In the following four decades, thousand of patients affected by end-stage renal failure have been successfully treated with living-donor kidney transplantation. The data generated have confirmed the safety of a healthy donor to donate one kidney in terms of physical performances and quality of life [6, 7]. Although safe and technically very successful, open nephrectomy is quite traumatic for the donor, and causes significant pain and discomfort. The consideration of the altruistic nature of kidney donation has motivated the transplant community to focus not only on avoiding potential surgical complications, but also on obtaining a rapid and complete restoration of donor health and physical fitness. Laparoscopic techniques were evaluated in the mid-1990s to achieve these goals.

Laparoscopic resection of diseased kidneys was first introduced by Clayman in 1991 [8]. Ratner et al. performed the first successful laparoscopic donor nephrectomy at John Hopkins University in 1995 [9]. Since then, the number of laparoscopic donor nephrectomies has rapidly grown, contributing greatly in increasing the number of living donor kidney transplants performed in the United States. Several centers have reported an increase in living-donor kidney transplants as high as 200% after the introduction of laparoscopic nephrectomy. In 2001, the number of living donors has exceeded the number of cadaveric donors for kidney transplantation for the first time, and the trend continues to date [2].

Although the technique originally described by Ratner has remained substantially unchanged in its fundamental steps, significant technological improvements have been added in the last few years.

One of the most important technical innovations has been the introduction of hand-assisted devices [10]. The introduction of the hand-assisted technique has determined a shortening of the learning curve and contributed to widespread application of laparoscopic donor nephrectomy. Commonly, the hand-assisted device is placed through an approximately 7 cm midline infraumbilical incision. The surgeon's arm is inserted into the LAP DISC hand port (Ethicon, Piscataway, N.J.) and used for manual retraction, dissection, hemostasis, and finally for kidney retrieval while maintaining pneumoperitoneum (while pneumoperitoneum is maintained by the special seal of the hand port).

The main advantages of the hand-assisted technique include improved ability to control bleeding vascular injuries, reduced length of surgery, and reduced warm ischemia time for the kidney graft [11].

In comparison with the open technique, laparoscopic nephrectomy has several recognized disadvantages, including increased operating room time, need for special equipment (usually quite costly), and limited ability of movement of the laparoscopic instruments, as well as two-dimensional (2D) rather than three-dimensional (3D) vision. In the attempt to improve the technical performance of laparoscopic donor nephrectomy, a program of robotic-assisted donor nephrectomy using the da Vinci® Robotic Surgical System was started in August 2000 (Intuitive Surgical, Sunny Valley, California).

Robotic surgery is a recent evolution of minimally invasive surgery aimed to obtain greater freedom of movement and to recreate the hand–eye coordination and 3D vision that is lost in standard laparoscopic procedures.

Technical details and various options currently available in robotic surgery are discussed in detail in Chap. 9.

The first robotic-assisted laparoscopic nephrectomy in a living human being was performed by Guillonneau et al. [12]. The authors reported a case of a right nephrectomy performed in a 77-year-old woman with a nonfunctioning, hydronephrotic right kidney, using the Zeus Robotic System.

In July 2000, the da Vinci® Robotic Surgical System was approved by the US Food and Drug Administration (FDA) for clinical use in the United States. The da Vinci® Robotic Surgical System combines robotics and computer imaging to enable microsurgery in a laparoscopic environment. The system consists of a surgeon's viewing and control console integrated with a high-performance, 3D monitor system and a patient side cart consisting of three robotic arms (Fig. 15.1).

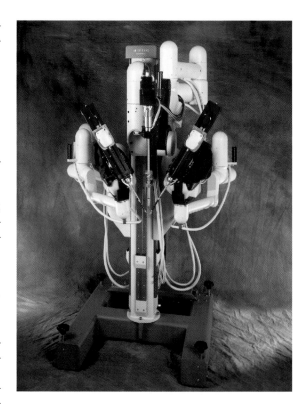

Fig. 15.1 Robotic arms

While observing the image of the operative field, the surgeon can control instrument movements via hand-controlled manipulators directly linked via electronics to motor-driven arms. These motor-driven arms hold and move instruments with standard surgical tool tips. The software within the da Vinci® Robotic Surgical System translates the surgeon's hand, wrist, and finger movements into corresponding micromovements within the patient's body, without any time delay. The instrument movements are under direct, real-time control of the surgeon. By using a kinematic structure (joint movement), the movements of the surgeon at the console are translated to the correspondent smaller instrument tip movements in the surgical field. The da Vinci® Robotic Surgical System provides the surgeon the benefits of access through small incisions without giving up the dexterity, precision, and instinctive movements of open surgery. Tip articulations mimic the up–down and side-to-side flexibility of the human wrist. These articulations extend the surgeon's minimally invasive abilities to a new level. In this system, the surgeon sits remote from the patient at an operating console adjusted to provide an optimal ergonomic environment.

In August 2000, our group successfully performed the first robotic-assisted donor nephrectomy for kidney transplantation with the da Vinci® Robotic Surgical System [13]. After a very favorable experience in a pilot study of 12 cases, we adopted robotic-assisted donor nephrectomy as our standard for living-donor kidney procurement. We discuss our current technique and the results to date below.

Between August 2000 and February 2004, we performed 112 robotic-assisted donor nephrectomies.

The donors were screened according to a thorough medical evaluation specified by a standardized protocol. Preoperatively, the donors underwent a spiral CT scan with 3D vascular reconstruction, which allows precise definition of the renal vascular anatomy.

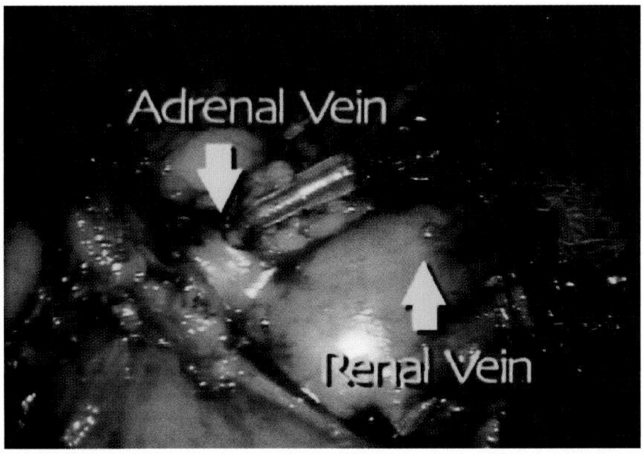

Fig. 15.3 Left renal vein

15.3   Surgical Technique

The donor nephrectomy is performed under general anesthesia, with the patient placed in the right decubitus position with pressure points padded. The operating table is flexed to maximize the exposure of the left kidney during the procedure. A 7-cm midline incision is performed immediately below the umbilicus, taken down through the fascia and into the abdominal cavity. A LAP DISC hand port is inserted, and pneumoperitoneum is achieved with 14 mmHg CO_2 insufflation.

Under direct visualization, a 12-mm trocar is placed at the level of the umbilicus on the left side of the abdominal wall, two 8-mm trocars are placed in the subxiphoid and left lower lateral abdomen, and another 12-mm trocar is placed in the left inguinal region. The da Vinci® Robotic Surgical System is then brought into position, and the arms are connected to the trocars.

The descending colon is freed from the lateral peritoneal attachments using electrocautery and reflected medially. The 3D view offered by the robotic system allows for a quick and safe identification of the ureter during dissection along the psoas (Fig. 15.2).

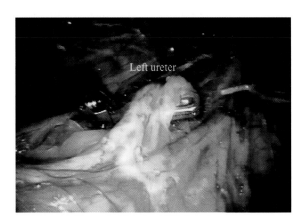

Fig. 15.2 Left ureter identification

The ureter is dissected free circumferentially in a cephalad direction, beginning at the level of the left common iliac artery. The posterior attachments of the kidney are then taken down. In this phase of the operation, the robot is particularly helpful in the dissection of the upper pole of the kidney from the retroperitoneal fat and the spleen, thanks to the articulated arm that reproduces the action of the human wrist.

The gonadal vein is identified medially and followed superiorly up to its junction with the left renal vein (Fig. 15.3).

The renal vein is then dissected free, and its tributaries (gonadal, lumbar and left adrenal veins) are divided between locking clips. At this point, the kidney is retracted medially and the main renal artery and any accessory renal artery are identified and dissected free up to the level of the aortic take-off.

The ureter is clipped twice distally at the level of the iliac artery and sharply transected. At this point, intravenous heparin at the dose of 80 units/kg is given. In the initial 60 cases, the renal artery was transected using a linear cutting vascular stapler (LCS, Ethicon). After experiencing three failures of the stapling device, resulting in conversion to open procedure, we modified the technique by first placing a locking clip (Hemo-Lok, Weck Closure Systems, Research Triangle Park, N.C.) at the take-off of the renal artery, and then dividing the artery with the stapling device. We used the stapling device alone for the transection of the renal vein in all cases. At this point, the left kidney is removed through the lower midline incision and taken to the back table where it is flushed with cold infusion of University of Wisconsin solution (ViaSpan™ Barr Laboratories, Pamona, N.Y.). Laparoscopic inspection of the renal bed is then performed to ensure hemostasis while intravenous protamine of appropriate dosage is administered. After evacuation of the pneumoperitoneum and removal of the trocars, the lower midline fascia is closed with a running no. 1 absorbable monofilament. The skin incisions are closed with subcuticular 4-0 absorbable monofilament and routinely infiltrated with 0.25% bupivacaine with epinephrine.

The robotic dissection of the left kidney with its vascular pedicle was successfully completed in all cases. However, in four cases conversion to open procedure was necessary because of abovementioned failure of the stapling device (three cases) and bleeding from renal vein laceration (one case). Mortality was 0%, while postoperative morbidity included pneumonia ($n = 1$), mild pancreatitis ($n = 1$), and superficial wound infections ($n = 3$), all successfully treated with conservative management. The mean hospital stay for robotic-assisted living-donor nephrectomy was comparable to standard and significantly shorter than was the open nephrectomy ($P = 0.05$).

The mean warm ischemia time was 79 s (ranging between 70 and 95 s).

The mean hospital stay decreased from 2.5 to 2.0 days, compared with standard laparoscopic donor nephrectomy. The patients were able to return to work after an average of 26 days (ranging from 12 to 49 days). All patients reported that although the laparoscopic approach did not influence their ultimate decision to donate a kidney, it did alleviate the anxiety surrounding their decision. One-year patient survival was 100%, while the 1-year graft survival was 98.8%. The incidence of delayed graft function was 0%. Two grafts were lost to acute rejection and renal thrombosis, respectively. We did not observe any urological complication. Average serum creatinine at 6 months posttransplant was 1.3 mg/dl.

In our experience, robotic-assisted donor nephrectomy has been an excellent tool to improve the safety and comfort of our living donors for kidney transplantation. Of course, experienced centers can obtain comparable results with pure laparoscopic techniques. However, the increased ability for a precise dissection and 3D visualization of the operative field provided by the robotic system is quite valuable. In the context of an advanced minimally invasive surgical center performing a large volume of complex laparoscopic procedures, the robot is becoming a critical component. If the transplant center operates in an institution supporting such a minimally invasive surgical center, it is logical and appropriate to use robotic technology to optimize living-donor care.

Furthermore, the robotic console is connected with the operating arms through cables. It is only a matter of improving the ability to transmit through cables the information before telerobotic surgery can be extensively applied. The advantages in terms of training and supporting peripheral centers in their effort to master complex operation would be invaluable.

15.4 Liver Transplantation

15.4.1 Technological Innovations in Transplant Surgery: from "Crash Clamp Technique" to Modern Instruments of "Intelligent" Dissection, Hemostasis

Fueled by the chronic scarcity of cadaveric donors, living-donor liver transplantation has become an accepted transplantation technique.

After the first attempts by Raia [14] and Strong [15] demonstrated the feasibility of the procedure, Broelsch in 1990 performed the first clinical series of living-related liver transplant in pediatric recipients [16, 17]. In the late 1990s, the procedure of living-donor liver transplant evolved from the left lateral hepatectomy for children to the more difficult and complicated prone right and left hepatectomy for adult patients.

Today, adult-to-adult living-donor liver transplantation is performed routinely in Europe, Asia, and the United States. Safety of the donor and the necessity of preserving the portion of the liver to be transplanted have totally changed the surgical approach to the hepatectomy. Vascular structures like the portal vein, the hepatic artery, the hepatic veins, and bile duct cannot just be ligated, but must be carefully dissected, preserved, and cut in order to provide intact vascular and biliary structures for the implantation. Complications that could be "accepted" in a patient undergoing hepatectomy for a liver tumor must be avoided in a healthy donor.

Consequently, the past 15 years have seen a tremendous effort to improve the surgical technique, especially the parenchymal transection of the liver with the aim of decreasing blood loss, operative time, complication incidence, and obtaining perfect vascular and biliary structures for the anastomosis in the recipient. Already in 1990, Broelsch wrote in relation to the complication incidence, "We think they can be prevented in future cases … by meticulous parenchymal transection." The parenchymal transection was at that time performed by a combination of "crash clamp technique," and the hemostasis was provided by monopolar coagulator and/or by sealing of the cut surfaces with fibrin glue. In the following decade, several technical innovations have made living liver donation safer and have modified the surgical approach to liver parenchymal transection. Living-donor liver transplantation is the only transplantation method in Japan and the Far East, and it is performed in 46 centers in Europe and in 56 centers in the United States [18]. In terms of results, the more recent data from European Liver Transplant Registry [19] show that survival of living-related liver transplantation in children is better than cadaveric liver transplantation. In adults, living-donor liver transplantation has the same patient and graft survival as cadaveric transplantation while assuring almost no primary nonfunction (4 vs. 8%, respectively) and fewer early retransplants of the liver (1 vs. 10%, respectively).

The confidence realized by many transplant surgeons in performing live-donor hepatectomy has allowed a broadening of the indications for the procedure, offering to many patients with previously untreatable conditions a chance for cure. An example of the expansion in indications is the patients affected by large hepatocellular carcinoma who now undergo living-donor liver transplantation [3–5, 20, 21]. It is paramount to perform the transection of the liver parenchyma, respecting all the anatomic vital structures and preventing any technical complication like bile leaks, bleeding, and vascular thrombosis. The transplant surgeon has many instruments that can be useful to obtain such an outcome. These instruments can be divided in three different groups: instruments that provide pure dissection, pure hemostasis and simultaneous dissection and hemostasis. The following describes their application in transplant surgery.

15.5   Transection Systems

15.5.1   Ultrasonic Dissector

The ultrasonic dissector does not possess hemostatic properties, but serves only to remove or divide parenchyma, exposing vascular structures and bile ducts. These structures can be then controlled with conventional technique (ligation, clipping, coagulation) or by the use of the harmonic scalpel. The ultrasonic vibration (range about 100 μ) of the hand piece hollow titanium tip selectively destroys liver parenchyma cells because of their high water content. It preserves the vascular and bile duct structures due to their higher content of elastin and collagen. The tip of the hand piece is constantly irrigated. A suction line parallel to the hollow tip aspirates the irrigation fluid, blood, and small tissue fragments. The ultrasonic dissector allows a decrease in blood loss and provides extensive exposure and dissection of large anatomical structures like portal and hepatic venous branches [22, 23]. Preservation of these structures is necessary when the resected portion of the liver will be used as a graft for the recipient.

15.5.2   Water-Jet Dissector

The water-jet dissector, or jet-cutter, is a device that like the ultrasonic dissector is able to produce a selective cutting action while discriminating between parenchyma and vascular and biliary structures [24, 25]. This instrument makes use of a high-pressure pump that imparts potential energy to a sterile saline fluid. Via a high-pressure line, the saline is conducted to a nozzle, from which it is delivered as a fine, high-pressure jet stream. By adjusting the pressure and nozzle parameters appropriately, it is possible to use such an instrument for selective cutting of the parenchyma. More resistant structures like veins, arteries, and bile ducts are left intact. Another important factor for the dissection of the parenchyma with the jet-cutter is the depth of penetration of the jet stream. This parameter is determined by pressure and nozzle size. In the pressure range of 60–80 bar, cutting is effective and practicable. There are at least three different systems of jet-cutter commercially available that differ in the accessories (handling or foot-pressure adjusting device) or in the type of pump (liquid-plus-gas or piston pump).

15.6   Hemostasis Systems

15.6.1   Staplers

The role of the staplers in open liver surgery was limited to division and stapling of large vessels previously dissected by other devices [26, 27]. The advantages are rapidity and relative safety of action. The application of the laparoscopic technique to liver surgery has familiarized surgeons with the use of the stapling device for transection of the liver parenchyma. The technique of stapling across the liver parenchyma allows an extremely fast and moderately bloodless parenchymal transection. The complete hemostasis on the cut surface of the liver can be obtained with a monopolar coagulator or/and a floating ball. Nevertheless, no data are available to determine whether this technique is safe also in preventing bile leaks in both the donor and the recipient.

15.6.2   Floating Ball

This technology combines a conductive fluid with radiofrequency energy. The conductive fluid is infused at the point of tissue contact by means of a ball at the end of the handheld device, while the thermal energy seals the tissue. By shrinking the natural collagen in the tissue, blood flow is stopped, and the tissue is sealed. While at the point of contact the temperature reaches 350°C, the fluid delivered at the tip of the handheld device cools the tissue and avoids the formation of eschar and tissue burning. The floating ball can coagulate vessels or ducts up to 10 mm in diameter. The major drawback in the use of this device in living donor hepatectomies is the spreading of the heat around the ball, which may cause damage to the vascular and biliary structures that must be left intact for the subsequent implantation [28].

15.7 Simultaneous Hemostasis and Transection

15.7.1 Thermal Methods

This group includes different instruments that have in common the ability to seal blood vessels or to cut surfaces by protein denaturation induced by heat. Among these instruments are the laser, the monopolar electrical cautery (Bovie) and the bipolar cautery. In the living-donor hepatectomy, only the monopolar and bipolar cauteries are frequently used. A popular technique is to use either instrument to obtain coagulation of small vessel on the cut surface of the parenchyma that has been previously transected with other devices, i.e., the ultrasonic or the water-jet dissectors [29].

15.7.2 Harmonic Scalpel

The harmonic scalpel represents one of the most innovative instruments introduced in the last decade, and is the only one that can practically combine dissection and hemostasis functions. The harmonic scalpel uses ultrasonic energy and eliminates the passage of electrical energy through the patient, like in conventional electrosurgery. The harmonic scalpel cuts and coagulates the tissue at temperature lower than 100°C. Cutting speed and coagulation are inversely related. More power results in increased distance traveled by the blade. Some devices are available with several power levels varying from a range of 50 to approximately 100 µm, which overall provide efficacious compromise between hemostasis and dissection in virtually any tissue encountered during surgery. The lower temperature and more controllable energy form result in smaller lateral thermal tissue damage.

Despite its characteristics, the harmonic scalpel has not found a consistent application in living-donor hepatectomy. One possible explanation might be that some investigators have not found any advantage in terms of transection speed, decreased blood loss, and decreased complications incidence when comparing the harmonic scalpel with the traditional crush clamp technique or the ultrasonic and water-jet dissectors [30, 31].

15.7.3 Laparoscopic Donor Hepatectomy for Living-Related Transplantation

The most exciting innovation in living-donor liver transplant surgery is the living–liver donor hepatectomy. The introduction of laparoscopy to living-related renal transplantation has tremendously increased the incentive to donate while maintaining excellent donor and recipient outcomes. It is foreseeable that a similar effect may be brought by the systematic utilization of laparoscopic surgery in the living donor hepatectomy.

The benefit of decreasing postoperative pain by replacing the large subcostal incision now utilized with a smaller lower abdominal incision is evident. On the other hand, many technical aspects must be solved before a routine application of laparoscopy will be possible.

At the present time only left lateral hepatectomy including segments 2 and 3 has been performed by laparoscopy [32– 36].

The operation described is based on a hand-assisted laparoscopic approach through a suprapubic incision and five trocars. Carbon dioxide is used for pneumoperitoneum, and the transection of the liver parenchyma is performed with the ultrasonic dissector and the harmonic scalpel. Hemostasis is obtained by bipolar electrocoagulation, and a vascular stapler is used for the control of the larger vessels. At the time of the writing of this chapter, there is no official report of a laparoscopic right or left hepatectomy for donation to an adult patient. Due to the great interest of the industry in creating new and safer technology for laparoscopic surgery and the to the growing confidence of many surgeons in laparoscopic liver resection, it is possible that in the next decade laparoscopic donor hepatectomy will be performed as routinely as laparoscopic donor nephrectomies.

References

1. Organ Procurement and Transplantation Network/United Network for Organ Sharing (2003) Organ Procurement and Transplantation Network/United Network for Organ Sharing (OPT/UNOS) data as December 2003. http://unos.org

2. US Department of Health and Human Services, Health Resources and Services Administration (2001) 2001 Annual report of the US Organ Procurement and Transplantation Network and the Scientific Registry for Transplants Recipients: Transplant Data 1991–2000. Rockville, Md.; US Department of Health and Human Services, Health Resources and Services Administration, Office of Special Programs, Division of Transplantation, Ann Arbor, Mich.; United Network for Organ Sharing: Richmond, Va.; University Renal Research and Education Association, Ann Arbor, Mich.

3. Bismuth H, Chice L, Adam R et al (1993) Liver resection versus transplantation for hepatocellular carcinoma in cirrhosis. Ann Surg 218:145–151

4. Iwatsuky S, Startzl TE, Sheahan DG, Yocoyama I et al (1991) Hepatic resection versus transplantation for hepatocellular carcinoma. Ann Surg 214:221–228

5. Roberts JP (2003) Role of adult living liver donation in patients with hepatocellular cancer. Liver Transpl 9(Suppl 2): S60–S63

6. Merlin TL, Scott DF, Rao MM et al (2000) The safety and efficacy of laparoscopic live-donor nephrectomy: a systematic review. Transplantation 70:1659

7. Brown SL, Biehl TR, Rawlins MC et al (2001) Laparoscopic live donor nephrectomy: a comparison with the conventional approach. J Urol Mar 165:766–769

8. Clayman RV, Kavoussi LR, Soper NJ et al (1991) Laparoscopic nephrectomy: initial case report. J Urol 146:278

9. Ratner LE, Buell JF, Kuo PC (2000) Laparoscopic donor nephrectomy: pro. Transplantation 70:1544

10. Wolf Stuart J Jr, Marcovich R, Merion R et al (2000) Prospective, case matched comparison of hand assisted laparoscopic and open surgical live donor nephrectomy. J Urol 163:1650–1653

11. Lindstrom P, Haggman W, Wadstrom J (2002) Hand-assisted laparoscopic surgery (HALS) for live donor nephrectomy is more time- and cost-effective than standard laparoscopic nephrectomy. Surg Endosc 16:422–425

12. Guillonneau B, Jayet C, Tewari A et al (2001) Robot-assisted laparoscopic nephrectomy. J Urol Jul 166:200–201

13. Horgan S, Vanuno D, Sileri P, Cicalese L, Benedetti E (2002) Robotic-assisted laparoscopic donor nephrectomy for kidney transplantation. Transplantation 73:1474–1479

14. Raia S, Nery JR, Mies S (1989) Liver transplantation from live donors. Lancet 2:497

15 Strong RW, Lynch SV, Ong TH, Matsunami H, Koido Y, Balderson GA (1990 Successful liver transplantation from a living donor to 1 son. N Engl J Med 322:1505–1507

16 Broelsch CE, Emond JC, Thistlethwaite JR, Whitington PF, Zucker AR, Baker AL, Aran PF, Rouch DA, Lichtor L (1988) Liver transplantation, including the concept of reduced-size liver transplants in children. Ann Surg 208:410

17. Broelsch CE, Emond JC, Whitington PF, Thistlethwaite JR, Baker AL, Lichtor L (1990) Application of reduced-size liver transplants as split grafts, auxiliary orthotopic grafts, and living related segmental transplants. Ann Surg 212:368–375

18. Based on Organ Procurement and Transplantation Network/United Network for Organ Sharing (2004) Based on Organ Procurement and Transplantation Network/United Network for Organ Sharing (OPT/UNOS) data as February 2004. http://unos.org

19. Ratner LE, Buell JF, Kuo PC (2002) Laparoscopic donor nephrectomy. Transplantation 70:1544; 73:1474–1479

20. Adam R, McMaster P, O'Grady JG, Castaing D et al (2003) Evolution of liver transplantation in Europe: report of the European Liver Transplant Registry. Liver Transpl 9:1231–1243

21. Bigourdan JM, Jaeck D, Meyer N, Meyer C, Oussoultzoglou E, Bachellier P et al (2003) Small hepatocellular carcinoma in Child A cirrhotic patients: hepatic resection versus transplantation. Liver Transpl 9:513–520

22. Koike Y, Shiratori Y, Sato S, Obi S, Teratani T, Imamura M et al (2000) Risk factors for recurring hepatocellular carcinoma differ according to infected hepatitis virus–An analysis of 236 consecutive patients with a single lesion. Hepatology 32:1216–1223

23. Yamamoto Y, Ikai I, Kume M et al (1999) New simple technique for hepatic parenchymal resection using a Cavitron Ultrasonic Surgical Aspirator and bipolar cautery equipped with a channel for water dripping. World J Surg 23:1032–1037

24. Putnam CW (1983) Techniques of ultrasonic dissection in resection of the liver. Surg Gynecol Obstet 157:474–478

25. Little JM, Hollands MJ (16991) Impact of the CUSA and operative ultrasound on hepatic resection. HPB Surg 3:271–277

26. Rau HG, Buttler ER, Baretton G et al (1997) Jet-cutting supported by high frequency current: new technique for hepatic surgery. World J Surg 21:254–259

27. Kaneko H, Otsuka Y, Takagi S et al (2004) Hepatic resection using stapling devices. Am J Surg 187:280–284

28. McEntee GB, Nagorney DM (1991) Use of vascular staplers in major hepatic resections. Br J Surg 78:40–41

29. Sakamoto Y, Yamamoto J, Kokudo N et al (2004) Bloodless liver resection using the monopolar floating ball plus ligature diathermy: preliminary results of 16 liver resections. World J Surg 28:166–172

30. Strasberg SM, Drebin JA, Linehan D (2002) Use of bipolar vessel-sealing device for parenchymal transection during liver surgery. J Gastrointest Surg 6:569–574

31. Kim J, Ahmad SA, Lowy AM (2003) Increased biliary fistulas after liver resection with the harmonic scalpel. Am Surg 69:815–819

32. Nakayama H, Masuda H, Shibata M et al (2003) Incidence of bile leakage after three types of hepatic parenchymal transection. Hepatogastroenterology 50:1517–1520

33. Cherqui D, Soubrane O, Husson E et al (2002) Laparoscopic living donor hepatectomy for liver transplantation in children. Lancet 359:392–396

34. Pinto PA, Montgomery RA, Ryan B et al (2003) Laparoscopic procurement model for living donor liver transplantation. Clin Transpl 17(Suppl 9):39–43

34. Kurian MS, Gagner M, Murakami Y et al (2002) Hand-assisted laparoscopic donor hepatectomy for living related transplantation in the porcine model. Surg Laparosc Endosc Percutan Tech 12:232–237

36. Lin E, Gonzalez R, Venkatesh KR et al (2003) Can current technology be integrated to facilitate laparoscopic living donor hepatectomy? Surg Endosc 17:750–753

Part V
Bioengineering

Tissue Engineering

16

Michael Shin and Joseph Vacanti

16.1 Introduction

Despite significant technological and medical advances, tissue loss and/or organ failure remains one of the most devastating and costly problems in health care. Since 1989, the number of patients has more than quadrupled in the United States alone. Currently, there are more than 80,000 patients on the national waiting list for organ transplants. In addition to this rapid increase, demand for donor organs continues to exceed supply by a substantial margin [1].

Currently, the most common treatment modalities include artificial devices, surgical reconstruction, and transplantation. In some instances, drug therapy is sufficient to replace the formation of metabolic products of a diseased or malfunctioning organ. This approach is common in endocrinology, and perhaps the best-known example is insulin injections for the treatment of diabetes. Improved delivery devices have resulted in better patient compliance, but the lack of normal feedback mechanisms may lead to an imbalance of hormonal levels and cause either acute or long-term complications [2, 3].

Artificial devices made of nonbiological materials, such as metals and plastics, are now routinely used in a variety of applications, ranging from joint replacements to mechanical heart valves and vascular grafts. These devices are also used in various extracorporeal applications such as dialysis. Due to the interface between the host tissue and the foreign material, artificial devices are prone to infection, thromboembolism, and frequently subject to limited materials durability [4]. The increased life expectancy of the aging population and the need for surgical treatments in increasing numbers of younger patients are placing greater demands on the durability and expected clinical lifetime of artificial prostheses. At present, well-designed prostheses have excellent clinical success rates for the first decade in most patients. However, in the second decade of the prosthesis' life, the failure rate and need for revision operations increase significantly [5, 6]. To alleviate these problems, research efforts are being undertaken to develop a better understanding of the behavior of materials in the physiological environment and thereby create more biocompatible and biomimetic materials [7–9]. While these research efforts are expected to lead to improved performance of artificial devices, the most important drawback of implantable artificial devices is the lack of growth potential, which is particularly relevant for pediatric patients.

Surgical reconstruction relies on using either different organs or unaffected tissue to replace damaged tissue or organs. Saphenous veins have been successfully used as bypass grafts. Myocutaneous flaps, either as pedicled flaps or as free tissue transfers, have also been effectively used for a variety of soft tissue defects [10–13]. However, since the replacement tissues are of a different tissue type, they are usually unable to restore full function. Furthermore, donor site morbidity and the scarcity of harvest sites remain critical issues [14].

Since the first successful transplant of the cornea in 1906, transplantation surgery has made significant advances [15]. The first successful human organ transplant was performed by Murray and colleagues in 1954, and the success with the kidney led to attempts with other organs [16–18]. Today, survival times ranging from 12 years (intestine) to more than 38 years (kidney) have been reported [19]. This success has been made possible by advances in transplantation biology and immunology, e.g., the introduction of tissue typing and the development of immunosuppressants to prevent allograft rejection. In particular, the discovery of cyclosporine brought transplants from research surgery to live-saving treatment [20, 21]. Despite these significant advances, organ and tissue transplantation remain imperfect solutions. Transplant recipients must follow lifelong immunosuppression regimes that are associated with increased risks of infection, potential for tumor development, and side effects. Most importantly, the aforementioned donor organ shortage limits the widespread availability.

To overcome these shortcomings, tissue engineering has been proposed as an alternative approach. The term *tissue engineering* was initially coined at a meeting sponsored by the National Science Foundation (NSF) in 1987. Formally, tissue engineering can be defined as "the application of the principles and methods of engineering and the life sciences toward the development of biological substitutes that restore, maintain or improve tissue function" [22]. Tissue engineering is an interdisciplinary approach that relies on the synergy of developmental biology, materials engineering, and surgery to achieve the goal of developing living substitutes that restore function and become fully integrated into the patient. Two principal approaches have been studied, the direct injections of selected cells, and combined transplantation of cells and biodegradable scaffolds to provide temporal structural support and guide tissue regeneration. The fundamental hypothesis underlying both approaches is that dissociated, healthy cells will reorganize into functional tissue when given the proper structural support and signaling cues.

Studies of direct cell injections have been carried out in animals and humans using a variety of cell types and organs [23–25]. This approach allows the use of selected cell populations to carry out a specific function and has attracted particular interest as a treatment option for infarcted myocardium [26, 27]. In addition, it is possible to manipulate cells prior to injection [24, 28, 29]. The injected cells rely on the stroma of the host organs for cell attachment and reorganization, and it is difficult to avoid migration of the injected cells.

The combination of temporary scaffolds and cells has become a key approach in tissue engineering (Fig. 16.1). Using this approach, tissue engineering requires three key components: (1) an appropriate cell source, (2) biodegradable scaffolds with suitable biological and mechanical properties, and (3) the proper environment to deliver the cells to the scaffold and promote attachment and proliferation.

Cells for tissue engineering may be drawn from a variety of sources. Primary cells may be autologous, syngeneic, allogeneic, or xenogeneic. The use of autologous or syngeneic cells is generally preferred to avoid immune reactions, but donor site morbidity or limited proliferative capability can be important limitations. At present, the use of allogeneic and xenogeneic cells is limited due to the need for host immunosuppression. Cell lines, i.e., cells that have been modified genetically to proliferate indefinitely, are attractive since they have the potential for rapid in vitro expansion and may be appropriate candidates for gene therapy. However, the tendency for cell lines to lose differentiated function and potential tumor formation are important con-

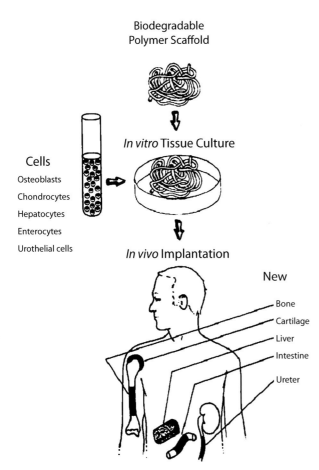

Fig. 16.1 Overview of the tissue engineering approach. Dissociated cells are harvested from an appropriate cell source and combined with a biodegradable, porous polymer scaffold that serves as a temporary extracellular matrix. Following an in vitro culturing period to increase cell attachment and proliferation, the constructs are implanted to replace or restore the function of missing tissue. (Reprinted with permission from [22])

cerns, and this requires further investigation. Recent advances in stem cell discovery have demonstrated the successful differentiation into various tissues like bone, cartilage, and muscle [30]. These discoveries have substantial potential for tissue engineering. Nonetheless, a more detailed understanding and control over differentiation is required to bring stem cells to clinical relevance.

The scaffold, typically in the form of a biodegradable polymer, serves several important functions. First, it acts as temporary filler for the defect site and prevents the formation of nonfunctional scar tissue. It also provides a temporary extracellular matrix (ECM) for the transplanted cells and guides tissue regeneration. Ideally, it also facilitates integration with the host tissue. The use of a scaffold provides better spatial control and permits the use of a higher cell number compared to injections alone. To this end, both natural and synthetic polymers have been investigated. Natural polymers, e.g., collagen, are appealing because they consist of ECM components and therefore mimic the native environment more closely. Since they are obtained from biological tissues, they are subject to batch-to-batch variations. Furthermore, there is concern about potential transmission of diseases. Synthetic polymers are very versatile materials because their chemical and physical properties can be tailored with a high degree of precision. The biocompatibility and degradation rate can be controlled during the polymer synthesis, and defined structures with appropriate mechanical properties can be fabricated reproducibly using a variety of polymer processing operations.

To obtain viable and functional tissue constructs from cells and biodegradable polymers, it is often necessary to culture the constructs in vitro for short period prior to implantation. Static culture conditions are usually sufficient to expand cells. However, to achieve optimal distribution, attachment, and proliferation of cells within the scaffold, a dynamic environment with appropriate mechanical forces, nutrient transfer, and gas exchange is required. The development of bioreactors in tissue engineering remains an active field of research. Various bioreactors have been developed to optimize the culture conditions through mixing, pulsatile flow and other mechanical stresses [31–33].

The remaining sections are organized as follows. Section 16.2 provides an overview of representative tissues and organs that have been investigated in tissue engineering. As representative examples, tissue-engineering approaches of skin, cartilage, bone, intestine, cardiovascular tissue, and liver are reviewed. The order of discussion reflects the increased complexity and challenges of regenerating quasi-two-dimensional and avascular tissues with low metabolic requirements to the regeneration of complex, vital organs. Section 16.3 describes the current shortcomings and the additional developments that are required to bring tissue engineering to widespread clinical reality. Future directions are also indicated. Section 16.4 addresses the relevance of tissue engineering for the practicing surgeon and concludes.

16.2 Overview

16.2.1 Skin

The skin is a highly organized, complex organ that consists of two principal outer layers, the epidermis and dermis. The epidermis is the outermost layer and protects the body from invasion and infection and helps to seal in moisture. It constantly proliferates and replaces itself. It does not contain any blood vessels, but instead obtains its oxygen and nutrients from the deeper layers of the skin. The dermis contains blood vessels, nerves, hair roots, and sweat glands. It is also rich in connective tissue that provides elasticity, firmness, and strength. The most important function of dermis is respiration. Wounds that extend only through the epidermis or partially through the dermis are capable of regeneration. If the wound extends through the entire thickness of the dermis, regeneration is no longer possible as there are no cell sources for regeneration. In cases such as full-thickness burns or deep ulcers, surgical solutions have been to apply autologous split-thickness skin grafts from uninjured sites or apply allogeneic grafts from cadaveric donors. Due to limited availability of donor sites or graft rejections, artificial skin has been pursued as a treatment for burn victims since the 1960s [34]. Since then, several strategies have been developed to create tissue-engineered skin, and three major approaches can be identified: (1) epidermal cells with no dermal layer; (2) only dermal layer; and (3) full-thickness graft, i.e., epidermis and dermis.

Epicel® is an epidermal autograft that consists of cultured keratinocytes on a polyurethane sheet. The polyurethane sheet acts as support for cell growth and application to the wound. Epicel® is grown from a patient's own skin cells and cocultured with mouse cells to form cultured epidermal autografts. Since the grafts are grown from autologous skin cells, they are not rejected by the patient's immune system. From a biopsy of healthy skin about the size of a postage stamp, enough skin can be grown to cover a patient's entire body surface in as little as 16 days. At present, Epicel® is the only permanent skin replacement product manufactured in the United States that is commercially available around the world. The shelf life of the grafts is 24 h, which enables the use of these grafts around the world. To date, more than 700 patients have been treated worldwide [35, 36].

Dermagraft® is the first tissue-engineered human fibroblast-derived allogeneic dermal substitute. In this approach, human foreskin-derived fibroblasts are grown on poly(lactide-co-glycolide) (PLGA) sheets. The fibroblasts proliferate to fill the interstices of this biodegradable scaffold and secrete human dermal collagen, matrix proteins, growth factors, and cytokines, to create a three-dimensional human dermal substitute containing living cells. These living skin substitutes are then cryopreserved until use. Dermagraft® has shown success in the treatment of diabetic foot ulcers [37, 38].

Apligraf® is a full-thickness graft that consists of allogeneic human keratinocytes and fibroblasts cultured on type 1 bovine collagen matrix. Like human skin, Apligraf® consists of two layers. The lower dermal layer combines bovine type 1 collagen and human fibroblasts (dermal cells) that produce additional matrix proteins. The upper epidermal layer is formed from human keratinocytes (epidermal cells) that replicate the architecture of the human epidermis. Apligraf® has been used in over 12,000 clinical and commercial applications, and is indicated for the treatment of venous leg ulcers and diabetic foot ulcers [39].

Skin was the first tissue-engineered organ to receive approval by the US Food and Drug Administration (FDA) for clinical applications, and is arguably the most successful example of tissue engineering to date. The aforementioned approaches, among others, have advanced from laboratory studies to clinical trials or commercial applications. Despite this success, there remain some concerns about the use of bovine-derived proteins and the possible risk of infection. Furthermore, tissue-engineered skin is currently limited to selected clinical applications and a truly universal tissue-engineered skin remains to be developed [40].

16.2.2 Cartilage

Cartilage is an avascular mesenchymal connective tissue that can be classified into three histological types—hyaline, elastic, and fibrous cartilage—that differ in contents and types of collagens, elastin, and proteoglycan matrix. Cartilage itself contains no blood vessels and obtains its blood supply from the overlying perichondrium. Due to the lack of blood supply and nervous innervation, it has a limited capacity for self-repair. In cases of small defects, cartilage is able to repair itself. However, in instances of partial or full-thickness defects, damaged cartilage cannot be repaired. Due to this limited self-repair potential and the low metabolic needs, cartilage is an attractive candidate for tissue engineering.

Initial studies demonstrated that primary chondrocytes that had been isolated from bovine cartilage could be seeded onto synthetic, biodegradable polymer scaffolds and produce neocartilage after transplantation into athymic mice [41]. Subsequent studies followed this pioneering approach by relying on FDA-approved poly(α-hydroxyesters) like polyglycolic acid (PGA), polylactic acid (PLA), and their copolymers (PLGA) as the scaffold. It was shown that cartilage could be generated in predetermined shapes using specially configured synthetic biodegradable polymer scaffolds (Fig. 16.2). The cartilage showed no signs of resorption or overgrowth throughout the entire experimental period. Histological examination confirmed the presence of normal mature hyaline cartilage [42]. Tissue-engineered cartilage was also successful in the treatment of surgically created cranial bone defects in a rat model [43]. Articular cartilage is of particular interest because full-thickness defects may progress to osteoarthritis. Using a rabbit model, new hyaline cartilage was created for resurfacing distal femoral joint surfaces that had been surgically denuded of articular cartilage. Evidence of new cartilage growth was found after 7 weeks, while animals in control groups showed virtually no new cartilage formation [44].

In addition to scaffold-based approaches, autologous chondrocyte transplantation without scaffolds has been used in a clinical study to repair deep cartilage defects in the femorotibial articular surface of the knee joint [45]. This has led to the development of Carticel®, consisting of autologous cultured chondrocytes, for the repair of symptomatic cartilage defects of the femoral condyle caused by acute or repetitive trauma in patients who have had an inadequate response to a prior arthroscopic or other surgical repair procedure. It should be mentioned that Carticel® is not indicated as a treatment for osteoarthritis. Here, a small biopsy of healthy knee cartilage is obtained and expanded in vitro. The cells are subsequently implanted under the periosteum in the defect and covered with a small piece of the periosteum to hold the cells in place. About 4,000 patients have been treated, and the results to date are promising.

In addition to creating cartilage in flat shapes, there have been significant efforts in creating complex, three-dimensional cartilage by using a variety of synthetic biodegradable polymers. Polymer templates in the form of nasoseptal implants were successfully used to guide the reorganization of bovine chondrocytes into neocartilage. All constructs showed evidence of formation of histologically organized hyaline cartilage [46]. A similar strategy was employed to create temporomandibular joint discs. The scaffolds maintained their specific shape, and histologically resembled hyaline cartilage. The mechanical properties were found to be similar to that of the native donor cartilage [47]. Cartilage formation was also successful in even more complex, three-dimensional architectures like the human

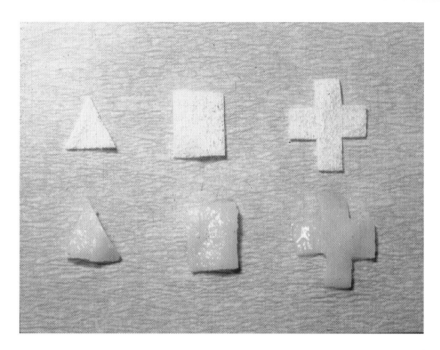

Fig. 16.2 Tissue-engineered cartilage in specific shapes. *Top row* Porous, nonwoven sheets of polyglycolic acid, an FDA-approved biodegradable polymer for biomedical applications. The polymer scaffolds were seeded with freshly isolated bovine articular chondrocytes and implanted subcutaneously into athymic mice. *Bottom row* Gross examination of the excised specimens 12 weeks after implantation revealed the presence of new hyaline cartilage of approximately the same dimensions as the original construct. (Reprinted with permission from [42])

ear [48, 49]. Significant efforts have also been undertaken to create a tissue-engineered trachea [50, 51]. A study using a sheep model demonstrated the feasibility of recreating the cartilage and fibrous portions of the trachea with autologous tissue harvested from a single procedure [52]. In addition, a methodology for creating a composite tracheal equivalent composed of cylindrical cartilaginous structures with lumens lined with nasal epithelial cells was developed [53]. These studies demonstrate the validity of the tissue-engineering approach, but important additional variables remain to be determined. The foremost question concerns the cell source. Since cartilage is found in various parts of the body, it is preferable to use a site for cell harvest that is easily accessible and requires less invasive methods. To this end, various cell sources have been assessed [54]. In addition, the effect of the cell age on proliferation and neocartilage formation was also investigated [55, 56].

In general, tissue-engineered cartilage has the histological appearance and biochemical composition of native cartilage. However, the mechanical strength of engineered cartilage is quite low. It has been shown that the aggregate modulus of tissue-engineered cartilage increases during the culture period, but the native tissue is still much stronger. Much of the mechanical properties of cartilage result from the interactions of negatively charged glycosaminoglycans and water. It is argued that without proper loading, chondrocytes may not produce sufficient amounts of proteoglycans, and the resulting cartilage lacks the impressive compressive strength of normal cartilage. Current efforts

are underway to develop bioreactors that improve the structure, function, and molecular properties of tissue-engineered cartilage [57, 58]. These efforts are likely to improve the long-term stability of tissue-engineered cartilage.

With the emergence of minimally invasive surgical techniques and improved diagnostic techniques, congenital malformations may be treated earlier. Several pilot studies in fetal tissue engineering have been undertaken, and the results are promising [59, 60]. In concert with these efforts, new scaffold materials are developed that allow delivery through small incisions and can fill irregularly shaped sites [61–63].

16.2.3 Bone

The treatment of bone defects remains a critical challenge in orthopedic surgery. Currently, bone grafts are used to treat defects caused by trauma, pathological degeneration, or congenital deformities. Bone grafting has become a common procedure in orthopedic surgery, and it is estimated that over 500,000 grafting procedures are performed each year in the United States [64]. Allografts are widely available and provide the defect site with structural stability. However, their use is limited by immunogenic response to foreign tissue, inflammation, and potential risk of disease transmission. Vascularized autografts show optimal skeletal incorporation and are currently considered the gold standard. However, important drawbacks are donor site morbidity and limited availability of donor sites. To over-come these problems, synthetic or natural biomaterials have been developed to promote the migration, pro-liferation, and differentiation of bone cells. Currently, several bone replacement materials are commercially available. These materials vary in composition and in-clude ceramics, polymers, and natural materials such as collagen and hydroxyapatite [65–67]. A common drawback of these materials is the lack of mechanical strength. Hence, their use is limited to bone void fill-ing applications. Furthermore, their potential to repair large bone defects is limited since they lack the osteo-conductive and osteoinductive properties of bone au-tografts. To date, there is no clinically available implant that mimics the function of living bone.

Tissue engineering offers the potential to create liv-ing bone in specific forms and shapes by combining a resorbable scaffold and suitable cells, leading to im-proved integration with the native bone and improved function. To achieve this goal, a variety of cell sources and scaffold materials have been assessed. Bovine peri-osteum-derived cells and degradable PGA fiber con-structs were successfully used to heal large segmental bone defects in the femurs of athymic rats. Histological evaluation revealed bone formation with islands of hy-pertrophying chondrocytes indicative of endochondral bone formation [68]. Phalanges and small joints were created by selective placement of bovine periosteum, chondrocytes, and tenocytes on biodegradable poly-

mer scaffolds and subsequent assembly into a compos-ite tissue structure (Fig. 16.3). Following implantation into athymic mice, mature articular cartilage and sub-chondral bone with a tenocapsule that had a structure similar to that of human phalanges and joints was ob-served [69]. Bone formation in heterotropic sites was also observed by injecting a mixture of fibrin glue and cultured periosteal cells into the subcutaneous space on the dorsum of athymic mice [70]. In a seminal clini-cal report, an avulsed phalanx of a patient was replaced with tissue-engineered bone. The procedure resulted in functional restoration of a stable thumb, without the pains usually associated with an autologous bone graft harvest [71].

Advances in stem cell biology have shown that the bone marrow contains regeneration-competent cells that can differentiate into osteoblasts, chondrocytes, ad-ipocytes, and myoblasts. These cells have been termed marrow stromal cells and are commonly referred to as mesenchymal stem cells (MSCs) [72–74]. Autologous bone marrow can be obtained conveniently from the iliac crest or sternum of a patient, using minimally in-vasive techniques with less pain and lower risk of infec-tion, hemorrhage, or nerve damage compared to bone graft harvests. Various studies have investigated bone formation from MSC-derived osteoblasts on biode-gradable polymer foams [75–79]. Typically, mineral-ization is observed within 2 weeks, but cell penetration and bone formation is limited to the outer sections

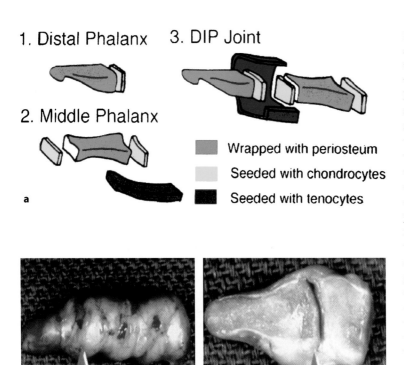

Fig. 16.3 Tissue-engineered phalanges and small joints. **a** Schematic represen-tation. Fresh bovine periosteum was wrapped around a copolymer of polyg-lycolic and poly-L-lactic acid. Separate sheets of polyglycolic acid polymer were seeded with bovine chondrocytes and tenocytes. The gross form of a composite tissue structure was constituted in vitro by assembling the parts and suturing them to create models of a distal phalanx, a mid-dle phalanx, and a distal interphalangeal joint. The sutured composite tissues were implanted into athymic mice. **b** After 20 weeks, formation of new tissue with the shape and dimensions of human phalan-ges with joints was observed. Histological examination revealed mature articular cartilage and subchondral bone with a tenocapsule that had a structure similar to that of human phalanges and joints. There was continuous cell differentiation at the ectopic site even after extended periods. (Reprinted with permission from [69])

of the scaffold. To address this problem and improve cell engraftment and survival, several approaches are currently being pursued. Scaffold fabrication techniques to create scaffolds with improved and more biomimetic architectures are being developed [80–83]. Mechanical stresses are important in determining the architecture of bone, and bioreactors are under development to provide the proper mechanical loading [84, 85]. An improved understanding of stem cell biology and in combination with gene therapy offers exciting potential to treat genetic disorders of skeletal tissues [86, 87]. It is expected that research activities in these areas will lead to the ultimate goal of bone tissue engineering, namely the development of vascularized bone grafts with clinically relevant dimensions.

16.2.4　Intestine

Digestive diseases affect more than 60 million Americans each year and account for more than $100 million in direct and indirect medical costs. Most digestive diseases are very complex and have subtle symptoms. In many cases, the cause(s) remain(s) unknown. Resection of the small intestine may be required, which can lead to a state of malnutrition and malabsorption if the functional gut mass is reduced below the minimum amount required for digestion and absorption to satisfy the nutrient and fluid requirements. This condition is commonly referred to as short bowel syndrome [88]. The normal physiologic process of intestinal adaptation after extensive resection usually allows for recovery of sufficient intestinal function within weeks to months, and during this time, patients can be sustained on total parenteral nutrition. However, prolonged parenteral nutrition can lead to complications such as hepatic dysfunction, progressive nephric insufficiency, and bone demineralization [89]. Surgical procedures such as small intestine tapering and lengthening have been undertaken to lengthen the bowel or increase intestinal transit time, but none have found widespread clinical application [90, 91]. Small intestinal transplantation is a promising surgical alternative, but the usual concerns regarding immunosuppression, rejection and limited donor supply remain [92].

Tissue engineering has been proposed as an alternative to allogeneic transplantation. In initial studies, enterocytes were isolated from neonatal Lewis rats, seeded on nonwoven PGA sheets, and formed into tubular structures. These constructs were implanted into the omentum or mesentery of syngeneic adult rats. Stratified epithelium was observed after 2 weeks, but the newly formed tissue had the histological appearance of embryonic intestine rather than adult intestine [93, 94]. It was hypothesized that this approach was limited due to the absence of epithelial–mesenchymal cell–cell interactions that are indispensable for survival, morphogenesis, proliferation, and differentiation. To allow for these interactions, the concept of epithelium organoid units was developed. These epithelium organoid units consist of a villus structure with overlying epithelium and a core of mesenchymal stromal cells. Mixed populations of enterocytes and stromal cells were harvested from the small intestine of neonatal Lewis rats, seeded on nonwoven PGA sheets, and transplanted into syngeneic adult rats. The epithelium organoid units maintained their epithelial–mesenchymal interactions and resulted in the formation of large cystic structures [95]. The inner lumen was lined with a neomucosa consisting of columnar epithelium containing goblet and Paneth cells, indicative of organ morphogenesis, cytodifferentiation, and phenotype maturation [96]. Subsequent studies showed that small bowel resection provides significant regenerative stimuli for morphogenesis and differentiation of tissue-engineered small intestine. Portacaval shunts were also stimulatory, but to a lesser extent [97, 98]. Implantation of the organoid unit/polymer constructs in highly vascularized beds such as the omentum or mesentery emerged as a reliable approach to form cystic structures with a small intestine-like morphology. The next step was to assess whether anastomosis between the tissue-engineered and native small intestine had an effect on cyst growth. Three weeks after implantation in the omentum, the tissue-engineered small intestine was anastomosed to the native jejunum in a side-to-side fashion. There was no evidence of stenosis or obstruction at the anastomosis site. Following anastomosis, the cysts were lined with a neomucosa that was continuous with the native small intestine across the anastomotic site. A positive effect of the anastomosis on the cyst size and the development of the mucosa in the tissue-engineered intestine were noted. Furthermore, crypt–villus structures were observed [99, 100]. Subsequent investigations to demonstrate the feasibility of end-to-end anastomoses showed a moderately high patency rate and a positive effect on the size of the neointestine and the development of the neomucosa [101]. Further studies were conducted to assess the effect of anastomosis alone or in combination with small bowel resection on neointestine organization [102]. A long-term investigation showed that anastomosis between tissue-engineered and native small intestine had a low complication rate after the operation and resulted in a high patency rate for up to 36 weeks. During this period, the neointestine increased in size and was lined with a well-developed mucosa [103].

The concept of epithelium organoid units was also applied to other organs of the gastrointestinal tract. A tissue-engineered colon was assessed as an alternative to an ileal pouch after a colectomy in a rat model. An end ileostomy alone was compared to an end ileostomy combined with a side-to-side ileum–tissue-engineered colon anastomosis. The tissue-engineered colon resulted in higher transit times, with lower stool moisture content and higher total serum bile acids [104]. The effect of cell source, i.e., adult or neonatal tissue, was also assessed. The architecture of the tissue-engineered colon resembles that of native colon (Fig. 16.4). Furthermore, it was found that the in vitro function was consistent with that of mature colonocytes [105].

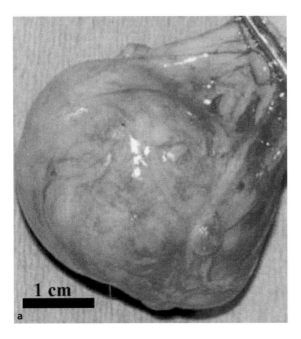

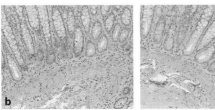

Fig. 16.4 a Gross morphology of tissue-engineered colon at 4 weeks after implantation in a rat model. Intestinal organoid units, mesenchymal cell cores surrounded by a polarized epithelia, were isolated from full-thickness sigmoid colon dissection, seeded on a polymer scaffold and implanted into the omentum of syngeneic hosts, resulting in cyst formation. The cysts were subsequently anastomosed to either the small or large intestine in a side-to-side fashion. **b** Immunohistochemical staining for actin of native (**a**) and tissue-engineered (**b**) colon. Both stain positively in the muscularis propria Original magnification ×10. (Reprinted with permission from [105])

The concept of a tissue-engineered stomach has also been investigated as an alternative to currently used reconstruction techniques after a total gastrectomy. Tissue-engineered stomachs were created from stomach organoid units isolated from neonatal and adult donor rats and implanted in syngeneic adult rats. The resulting cysts resembled native stomachs histologically [106]. Tissue-engineered stomachs were successfully used as replacement stomachs in a rat model by resecting the native stomach and anastomosing the tissue-engineered stomach between the native esophagus and jejunum. An upper gastrointestinal study revealed no evidence of bowel stenosis or obstruction at both anastomosis sites. Histologically, the tissue-engineered stomachs had well-developed, vascularized tissue with a neomucosa continuously lining the lumen and stratified smooth muscle layers [107].

Tissue engineering of the gastrointestinal tract has been shown to be a versatile model for studying the gastric physiology. Using this approach, important insights into tissue development and potential therapy can be gained. A recent study has characterized the microvasculature and angiogenic growth factor profile of tissue-engineered intestine. While tissue-engineered intestine has the histological appearance of native tissue, the mechanism driving angiogenesis differs in tissue-engineered intestine and in normal small intestine. Delivery of angiogenic factors like vascular endothelial growth factor (VEGF) and basic fibroblast growth factor (bFGF) is proposed as a remedy, and this may bring tissue-engineered intestine closer to clinical applications [108].

16.2.5 Cardiovascular Tissue

Atherosclerotic vascular disease remains a leading cause of mortality and morbidity in industrialized nations. Autologous veins are the conduits of choice in the surgical creation of bypasses of short- to medium-caliber vessels in patients with peripheral occlusive arterial disease. The success rate of bypasses using conduits with diameters greater than 6 mm has been excellent, whereas the majority of bypasses using smaller conduits typically fail within 5 years. Furthermore, suitable donor sites are limited. Allogeneic grafts carry the risk of rejection and potential disease transmission, though there is recent evidence that autologous cells seeded on decellularized allogeneic vessels may provide a suitable alternative [109]. Artificial grafts face similar drawbacks in that they work reasonably well for large diameter grafts, but they have a high failure rate in small diameter grafts. Furthermore, there is a potential for infection and thrombosis. Reoperations may also be required due to calcification [110].

Due to these limitations, tissue engineering of blood vessel substitutes has become an active area of research. Early attempts focused on the creation of hybrid grafts by attempting to line the lumen of artificial graft materials with endothelial cells [111]. Subsequently, many different approaches have been taken, relying on both synthetic and natural scaffolds. A multilayered blood vessel was created in vitro by combining smooth muscle cells in collagen gel, fibroblasts, and endothelial cells. Although the histology resembled that of an artery, the mechanical properties were not sufficient for the systemic circulation [112]. A scaffold-free approach using human cultured cells resulted in increased burst strength, but the patency rate was only 50% over 7 days in an animal model [113]. A small-diameter, tissue-engineered vessel was created from small intestinal submucosa and showed excellent hemostasis and patency in a rabbit arterial bypass model. Within 3 months after implantation, the grafts were remodeled into cellularized vessels that exhibited physiological activity in response to vasoactive agents [114]. Following the use of natural scaffolds, the use of synthetic biodegradable scaffold was assessed in a seminal study to create tissue-engineered arteries. In addition, a pulsatile flow bioreactor was used to create a more physiological environment and improve the mechanical strength of the graft. The tissue-engineered graft had the histological appearance of a native artery and was able to sustain systemic pressures. The tissue-engineered arteries were implanted in a pig model and remained patent for up to 4 weeks [115].

Repair of congenital cardiac defects frequently require large diameter conduits. As stated earlier, artificial grafts are now routinely used. However, due to the lack of growth potential, they are not suitable for pediatric patients. Viable pulmonary arteries were created by seeding cells derived from ovine artery and vein segments onto synthetic biodegradable PGA/PLGA scaffolds in tubular shape. These autologous constructs were used to replace a 2-cm segment of the pulmonary artery in lambs. All tissue-engineered grafts were patent and demonstrated a non-aneurysmal increase in diameter, suggesting growth [116]. A similar methodology was applied to replace a 3- to 4-cm segment of the abdominal aorta in lambs. Here, a new copolymer of PGA and polyhydroxyalkanoate (PHA) was combined with cells harvested from ovine carotid arteries. All tissue-engineered grafts remained patent, and no aneurysms had developed over a course of 3 months. Histologically, elastic fibers were observed in the medial layer, and endothelial cells lined the lumen. Furthermore, the mechanical properties of the tissue-engineered aorta approached those of the native vessel. In addition to full segment replacements, patch augmentation of vessels has also been investigated. Vascular cells isolated from ovine peripheral veins were seeded

on a fast-absorbing biopolymer, poly-4-hydroxybutyric acid (P4HB), and assessed for patch augmentation of the proximal pulmonary artery in a juvenile sheep model. Postoperative echocardiography showed no signs of dilatation or stenosis. Macroscopically, a smooth internal surface with increasing tissue formation was observed [117]. Another study demonstrated the successful replacement of the inferior vena cava in a dog model. In this approach, mixed cells obtained from the femoral veins of mongrel dogs were seeded onto tube-shaped biodegradable polymer scaffolds composed of a PGA nonwoven sheet and a polycaprolactone-polylactide copolymer (PCLA). No implants showed evidence of dilatation or stenosis. In addition, an endothelial lining was observed in all tissue-engineered grafts [118].

An important milestone for tissue engineering was achieved in May 2000, when an occluded pulmonary artery was successfully replaced by a tissue-engineered graft in a 4-year-old girl with a single ventricle and pulmonary atresia that had previously undergone pulmonary artery angioplasty and the Fontan procedure. Following harvest of a short segment of peripheral vein, cells were isolated, cultured in vitro and seeded on a tubular PCLA scaffold. Ten days after seeding, the graft was transplanted. Seven months after implantation, the patient was doing well. Chest radiography revealed no evidence of graft occlusion or aneurysmal changes [119]. The same methodology was applied in a subsequent case to replace an occluded Dacron graft in the extracardiac Fontan operation (ECFO) of a 12-year-old boy. The reoperative ECFO with a tissue-engineered graft was successful, and postoperative computed tomography done 4 months after the operation revealed a patent graft [120]. Subsequently, aspirated bone marrow cells were used as the cell source and seeded on the scaffold on the day of surgery. Using this method, sufficient cells could be obtained on the day of the surgery without requiring a culturing period. Furthermore, extra hospitalization for vein harvesting is not required. This approach has been applied in 22 patients, and good results were obtained after surgery [121]. The contribution of bone marrow cells to the histogenesis of autologous tissue-engineered vascular grafts was also demonstrated [122]. In addition, a new technique of extracardiac total cavopulmonary connection using a tissue-engineered graft has been developed, and the initial results are promising (Fig. 16.5) [123].

Tissue-engineered vascular grafts have shown promise in the aforementioned complicated cases. It is anticipated that their indications will be increased for other types of cases. While the initial clinical success is very promising, there remain limitations of this method in a clinical setting. First, these tissue-engineered grafts are currently limited to the pulmonary circulation. Tissue-engineered grafts cannot be used in the systemic

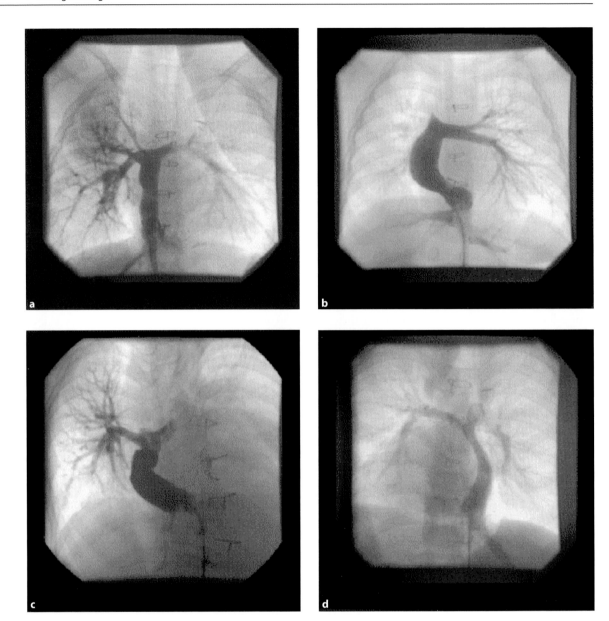

Fig. 16.5 Angiograms of tissue-engineered grafts 6 months after undergoing an extracardiac total cavopulmonary connection (TCPC) operation in Patient 2 (**a**), 4 months after TCPC in Patient 3 (**b**), 1 month after TCPC in Patient 4 (**c**), and 8 months after TCPC in Patient 6 (**d**). Note the smooth surface of the tissue-engineered graft and well-enhanced pulmonary arteries. (Reprinted with permission from [123])

circulation due to the higher pressures and flow velocities. To achieve this goal, further development of biodegradable scaffolds is required. Second, a tissue-engineered graft cannot be used in an emergency operation due to the prolonged in vitro period necessary for cell engraftment on the scaffold. Third, a sufficient cell number may not be available in all patients. In such cases, additional cell sources from other parts of the body must be assessed. Active research continues

in this field to overcome these challenges. Efforts are devoted to modifying the culture environment to enhance extracellular matrix synthesis and organization using bioreactors under physiologic conditions and biochemical supplements. Improved understanding of the factors involved in cardiovascular development and advances in gene therapy and stem cell biology are also expected to contribute toward the goal of widespread clinical applications.

16.2.6 Liver

The field of liver regeneration and liver support remains one of the most complex and unsolved medical problems. According to the American Liver Foundation, 25 million Americans suffer from liver and biliary diseases. In 1993, liver disease became the seventh leading cause of death in the United States, and each year, about 30,000 people die from end-stage liver failure. There are currently few effective treatments for severe liver diseases. In contrast to other end-stage organ failures, liver transplantation is the only established successful treatment for liver failure. Again, the discrepancy between supply and demand of organs is staggering. It is estimated that approximately 5,000 liver transplants were performed in 2000. However, almost 1,700 prospective recipients died in 2001 while waiting for a liver for transplantation. At present, there are over 18,000 people waiting for a liver transplant [124].

In efforts to overcome the severe donor organ shortage, several alternative therapies have been explored. These include split liver cadaveric grafts, living donor transplants, xenografts, and selected cell transplantations [125–130]. Several approaches have also been developed for the transplantation of hepatocytes. Direct injections of cell suspensions have been carried out in a variety of locations such as the liver, spleen, or pancreas [131–133]. In addition, approaches involving encapsulations or microcarrier beads have also been assessed [134, 135]. Transplanted hepatocytes were able to maintain normal hepatocellular architecture and demonstrated functional ability for a limited time. However, it has been difficult to achieve a sufficient cell mass to replace lost function.

The difficulty of liver regeneration stems in part from the vast complexity of the tissue. The liver is the largest internal organ and consists of several cell types arranged in a highly complex architecture. It is highly vascularized and performs a large number of metabolic functions. Hepatocytes, the major liver cell type, are anchorage-dependent cells and require an insoluble extracellular matrix for survival, reorganization, proliferation, and function. In addition, they are highly metabolic cells and require close proximity to nutrient and oxygen supply. To achieve a higher cell number and structural support for hepatocytes, hepatocyte transplantation combined with synthetic, highly porous, biodegradable scaffolds was proposed. Initial studies demonstrated the survival of transplanted hepatocytes on porous, biodegradable polymer disks in a peripheral site and in the small intestine mesentery in rats [136, 137]. Transplanted hepatocytes expressed liver-specific functions and survived for extended periods. However, a significant decrease in cell number was noted after transplantation.

To improve cell viability, a new approach exploring prevascularization was pursued. Empty scaffolds were placed between the leaves of the mesentery or subcutaneous pockets to promote fibrovascular ingrowth prior to cell injection. This led to improved cell engraftment and survival, but a large number of cells were lost within a week [138, 139]. Further improvement in cell engraftment and growth was achieved by considering the self-regulation of liver mass, i.e., transplanted livers will grow or atrophy to reach an appropriate size for the recipient. It was conjectured that transplanted hepatocytes were actively suppressed in the recipient due to the presence of a healthy native liver. To assess this conjecture, recipient animals underwent partial hepatectomies or portacaval shunts, resulting in an increased delivery of hepatotrophic factors to the systemic circulation and reduced clearance by the native liver. It was shown that hepatotrophic stimulation led to a significant improvement in cell survival [140–143]. Using this approach, a mass of Wistar rat hepatocytes equivalent to a whole liver was transplanted in Gunn rats, which have a genetic deficiency of glucuronyl transferase activity, showing unconjugated hyperbilirubinemia. Over a course of several weeks, a decrease in serum bilirubin levels was observed [144, 145]. The methodology of combined cell/polymer transplantation and surgical hepatotrophic stimulation has also been extended to large animals [146–148]. Another approach to overcome the insufficient engraftment has been to improve vascularization by local delivery of angiogenic factors. In one study, bFGF was incorporated into degradable scaffold, and increased angiogenesis and hepatocyte engraftment were observed [149]. A recent approach to overcome the critical limits of nutrient and oxygen diffusion has been the development of polymer scaffolds that can be implanted directly into the bloodstream [150]. Hepatocytes were dynamically seeded onto these scaffolds and placed in a flow reactor. The engrafted hepatocytes showed excellent survival with a high rate of albumin synthesis [151, 152].

A novel approach is the creation of a scaffold with an integrated vascular network to provide immediate access to the blood supply after implantation. A versatile scaffold fabrication method termed three-dimensional printing (3DP) offering unprecedented control over the geometry and architecture including controlled porosity and ingrowth channels was used to create complex three-dimensional biodegradable scaffolds [153]. Hepatocytes attached to the scaffold and survived under dynamic culture conditions in vitro. Albumin synthesis was demonstrated, and the hepatocytes reorganized into histotypical structures in the channels of the scaffold [154, 155]. The concept of prevascularization to provide improved cell engraftment and mass transfer of oxygen and nutrients was recently further refined through the adaptation of silicon microfabrication. This methodology is based on semiconductor wafer process technology originally developed for integrated circuits (IC) and microelectromechanical systems (MEMS). Silicon microfabrication offers submicron-scale resolution over several orders of magnitude from 0.1 mm to tens of centimeters [156]. Since this range covers the relevant physiological length scales from capillaries to large vessels, a concept was developed to create a complete branching vascular circulation in two dimensions on silicon wafers and subsequently build up three-dimensional structures by stacking or rolling. In a first demonstration, hepatocytes and endothelial cells were cultured on silicon and Pyrex wafers patterned with trenches reminiscent of a vasculature. Hepatocyte sheets were lifted off, folded into compact three-dimensional configurations, and implanted into rat omenta. This resulted in the formation of vascularized hepatic tissue [157]. Subsequent advanced have been the development of a computational model to create tissue-specific vascular networks and the transfer of this methodology to biocompatible polymers [158, 159]. Current research is in progress to transfer the process methodology to biodegradable polymers to arrive at the ultimate goal of thick, vascularized tissue-engineered organs (Fig. 16.6).

16.3 Future Prospects

The field of tissue engineering has reached a critical junction. The fundamental principles of tissue engineering are based on cell transplantation, which has been studied for more than 60 years. The concept of tissue engineering is appealing and easily understood by clinicians, scientists, investors, and the general public. During the 1990s, tissue engineering received highly favorable media attention. Tissue engineering was hailed as one of the greatest scientific achievements of the twentieth century, and both scientific and general media endorsed the field's potential. In 2000, *Time* magazine predicted that a career in tissue engineering would become one of the "10 Hottest Jobs of the Future" [160]. In 2002, *Science* magazine featured a special issue on the bionic human and the development of "off-the-shelf replacement parts for the human body" [161]. During the economic boom of the 1990s, there was significant capital inflow into tissue engineering, and several tissue-engineering companies were founded.

Twenty years later, the future seems to look less promising. Although the concepts have been known for 20 years, and serious research activity has been conducted for 15 years, there are only a few clinical applications of tissue engineering. An ambitious plan to grow a fully functioning heart from a Petri dish of human cells within 10 years was proposed by the LIFE (Living Implants From Engineering) initiative, based at the University of Toronto, and ultimately collapsed. Furthermore, the financial performance of companies with tissue-engineered products has been rather dismal, and almost all tissue-engineering companies have disappeared. The financial collapse of Advanced Tissue Sciences and Organogenesis, two of the leading tissue-engineering companies, is related to the economic recession, but also indicates decreased investor confidence. Currently, four products have received FDA approval. Apligraf®, Dermagraft®, and OrCel® are living-skin equivalents for the diabetic and venous ulcers and burn patients, and Carticel® consists of autologous chondrocytes for cartilage repair. In addition, ten tissue-engineered products are engaged in clinical trials, while another six products failed to meet efficacy in phase III or were abandoned during phases I or II. To assess the past performance and future of tissue engineering, it is important to distinguish between the scientific and finance-related aspects. A detailed discussion about the past performance and the economic lessons is beyond the scope of this chapter, and the interested reader is referred elsewhere [162].

Despite the failure of tissue engineering to grow whole, complex organs in the laboratory, the field is adapting and continuing to move forward. It has become apparent that the task of growing a whole organ is too complex, and a recent shift in focus toward individual components has occurred. One of the largest efforts is the BEAT (BioEngineered Autologous Tissue) initiative, based at the University of Washington and supported by a $10 million, 5-year grant from the National Institutes of Health (NIH) to create patches of cardiac muscle to repair the damage caused by heart attacks. Should this approach be successful, the next goal is to create a ventricle. This approach could possibly lead to a complete tissue-engineered heart. Hence, the concept of whole organs has not been completely abandoned yet. To achieve this goal, an even more integrated and interdisciplinary approach combining the life sciences, engineering and clinical medicine will be required.

One of the key limitations to applying cell-based therapies toward organ replacement has been the inherent difficulty to grow specific cell types in sufficient quantities. Even organs like the liver that have high regenerative capabilities in vivo, show reduced cell growth and expansion in vitro. The arguably greatest contribution for tissue engineering is from cell biology. The completion of the Human Genome Project is providing a wealth of information that is expected to lead to a more complete understanding of cells and cell behavior. Another critical contribution is the understanding of cell phenotype. The discovery of nuclear

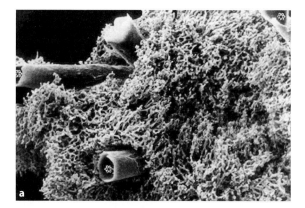

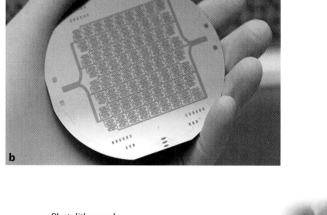

Fig. 16.6 a Vasculature of a human liver. Nature solves the mass transport problem by providing a convective network of blood vessels. The *asterisks* (*) denote the largest vessels, which subsequently branch into 10 generations of smaller vessels. (Reprinted with permission from Vonnahme FJ (1993). The human liver: a scanning electron microscopic atlas. Karger, Basel). **b** Silicon microfabrication offers enhanced resolution to create a network of channels with a topology reminiscent of a vasculature. The network design is created using a computational model that mimics blood flow and takes blood rheology into account. Silicon wafers with etched channels are created using standard microfabrication techniques. **c** Schematic representation of the microfabrication approach to create vascularized tissue-engineered organs. (Reprinted with permission from IEEE Spectrum Online, http://www.spectrum.ieee.org)

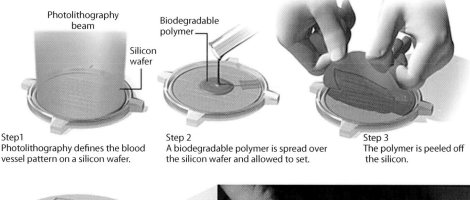

Step 1
Photolithography defines the blood vessel pattern on a silicon wafer.

Step 2
A biodegradable polymer is spread over the silicon wafer and allowed to set.

Step 3
The polymer is peeled off the silicon.

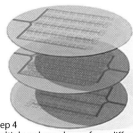

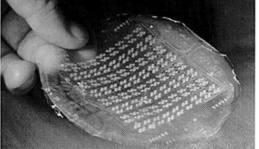

Step 4
Multiple polymer layers from different molds are joined to form the scaffold for the engineered organ.

c

transfer has shown that reprogramming nuclear DNA to express many phenotypic programs is possible. It is anticipated that this will lead to a better understanding of differentiation pathways. Adult and embryonic stem cells have also become the focus of attention due to their inherent plasticity. Embryonic stem cells are of particular interest because they can be expanded in an undifferentiated state in vitro and subsequently induced to form many different cell types. This is particularly beneficial in applications where the source of cells is limited or not available. Stem cell research and gene therapy are still in the early stages, so their full biology and therapeutic potential remain to be discovered. Other areas of interest are wound healing and tissue assembly. While cell biology has traditionally focused on molecular events on a cellular level, efforts to move to the next hierarchical level and understand how molecules and cells form tissues will directly contribute to tissue engineering. Cancer research is another area that is likely to affect tissue engineering because the formation of blood vessels is central to both fields [163].

Another active area of research is biomaterials and scaffold development. Since the early days of using debrided surgical sutures as a scaffold, materials synthesis and processing have made significant advances. New fabrication methods for creating three-dimensional scaffolds with improved mechanical properties and surface chemistries have emerged. Integration with imaging and the development of patient-specific scaffolds is also actively investigated [154]. New materials are being synthesized, e.g., biomimetic natural and synthetic polymers, and osteoconductive ceramics [164–166]. A detailed understanding of cell–material interactions is also crucial. The ultimate goal is to create scaffolds that encode specific instructions for controlling tissue formation, analogous to signals during embryological development. The biggest challenge is the creation of three-dimensional structures that contain more than several cell layers. To this end, several approaches have emerged. The incorporation of growth factors to induce angiogenesis is one strategy that is showing promise [167, 168]. However, angiogenesis takes 3 to 5 days, and this approach may be limited to specific applications. Another approach is to abandon the scaffold and stack individual cell layers. This versatile approach has been applied to many different tissues and has significant potential [169]. Advances in active research areas such as nanotechnology, hydrogels, and self-assembled materials are also expected to find application in tissue engineering [170–172].

Despite the initial problems, tissue engineering has a bright future. The overall goal of tissue engineering of developing tissue equivalents for the repair, replacement, maintenance, or augmentation of tissue and organs is expected to have a significant impact on health care. However, the impact of tissue engineering

is expected to be even more significant. In addition to *therapeutic* tissue engineering as discussed here, *diagnostic* tissue engineering is emerging as an approach to develop tissue equivalents for in vitro drug testing and the development of improved therapeutic agents. In particular, the development of human tissue equivalents would alleviate some of the problems associated with species-specific events. If the tissue is organized in its native configuration rather than in a two-dimensional Petri dish, such constructs are expected to be better models for the search of therapeutic treatments and improve the physiologic relevance of in vitro testing.

16.4   Relevance for the Practicing Surgeon

Although tissue engineering is far from being a widely applied clinical treatment, the field has taken steps closer toward clinical applications. With the recent shift of research efforts beyond the United States to Europe and Asia, the number of clinical studies has increased significantly. In addition to the clinically approved tissue-engineered skin and cartilage products, several promising clinical studies are currently in progress. The replacement of a human phalanx by a tissue-engineered construct showed good results, but generated questions about the therapeutic value and improvement compared with conventional treatments [71]. This discussion indicates that tissue engineering is not the solution to every medical problem requiring tissue replacement. Tissue engineering must be seen within the context of present-day medicine. Clinical applications must be chosen carefully and compared critically to existing treatment modalities. In addition to bone, urological tissue is in the early stages of clinical application [173]. The perhaps most advanced clinical trials are currently being conducted in Japan, and the promising results are indicative of the clinical potential of tissue engineering. The clinical success of tissue engineering will require an interdisciplinary approach and depend critically on continued collaborations between engineers, scientists, and clinicians.

References

1. UNOS Annual Report of the US Scientific Registry of Transplant Recipients and the Organ Procurement and Transplantation Network (2006) http://www.unos.org
2. Korytkowski M, Bell D, Jacobsen C, Suwannasari R, Team FS (2003) A multicenter, randomized, open-label, comparative, two-period crossover trial of preference, efficacy, and safety profiles of a prefilled, disposable pen and conventional vial/syringe for insulin injection in patients with type 1 or 2 diabetes mellitus. Clin Ther 25:2836–2848

3. Hermansen K, Ronnemaa T, Petersen AH, Bellaire S, Adamson U (2004) Intensive therapy with inhaled insulin via the AERx insulin diabetes management system: a 12-week proof-of-concept trial in patients with type 2 diabetes. Diabetes Care 27:162–167

4. Hench LL, Ethridge EC (1982) Biomaterials: an interfacial approach. Academic Press, New York

5. Ikonomidis JS, Kratz JM, Crumbley A Jr, Stroud MR, Bradley SM, Sade RM, Crawford FAJ (2003) Twenty-year experience with the St Jude Medical mechanical valve prosthesis. J Thorac Cardiovasc Surg 126:2022–2031

6. Jacobs JJ, Hallab NJ, Skipor AK, Urban RM (2003) Metal degradation products: a cause for concern in metal-metal bearings? Clin Orthop 417:139–147

7. Sagnella S, Kligman F, Marchant RE, Kottke-Marchant K (2003) Biometric surfactant polymers designed for shear-stable endothelialization on biomaterials. J Biomed Mater Res 67A:689–701

8. Sarikaya M, Tamerler C, Jen AK, Schulten K, Baneyx F (2003) Molecular biomimetics: nanotechnology through biology. Nat Mater 2:577–585

9. Shin H, Jo S, Mikos AG (2003) Biomimetic materials for tissue engineering. Biomaterials 24:4353–4364

10. Kouchoukos NT, Karp RB, Oberman A, Russell ROJ, Alison HW, Holt JHJ (1978) Long-term patency of saphenous veins for coronary bypass grafting. Circulation 58: I96–I99

11. Chapelier AR, Missana MC, Couturaud B, Fadel E, Fabre D, Mussot S, Pouillart P, Dartevelle PG (2004) Sternal resection and reconstruction for primary malignant tumors. Ann Thorac Surg 77:1001–1006; discussion, 1006–1007

12. Klinkert P, Post PP, Breslau PP, Van Bockel JJ (2004) Saphenous vein versus PTFE for above-knee femoropopliteal bypass: a review of the literature. Eur J Vasc Endovasc Surg 27:357–362

13. Yamamoto Y, Kawashima K, Sugihara T, Nohira K, Furuta Y, Fukuda S (2004) Surgical management of maxillectomy defects based on the concept of buttress reconstruction. Head Neck 26:247–256

14. Mont MA, Etienne G, Ragland PS (2003) Outcome of nonvascularized bone grafting for osteonecrosis of the femoral head. Clin Orthop 417:84–92

15. Zirm EK (1989) Eine erfolgreiche totale Keratoplastik [A successful total keratoplasty]. 1906. Refract Corneal Surg 5:258–261

16. Murray JE, Merrill JP, Harrison JH (1955) Renal homotransplantation in identical twins. Surg Forum 6:432–436

17. Starzl TE (2001) The birth of clinical organ transplantation. J Am Coll Surg 192:431–446

18. Starzl TE (2003) Organ transplantation: a practical triumph and epistemologic collapse. Proc Am Philos Soc 147:226–245

19. Cecka JM, Terasaki PI (2001) Clinical transplants. UCLA Immunogenetics Center, Los Angeles

20. Patel JK, Kobashigawa JA (2004) Cardiac transplant experience with cyclosporine. Transplant Proc 36:S323–S330

21. Zuckermann A, Klepetko W (2004) Use of cyclosporine in thoracic transplantation. Transplant Proc 36:S331–S336

22. Langer R, Vacanti JP (1993) Tissue engineering. Science 260:920–926

23. Mito M, Ebata H, Kusano M, Onishi T, Saito T, Sakamoto S (1979) Morphology and function of isolated hepatocytes transplanted into rat spleen. Transplantation 28:499–505

24. Kodama S, Kuhtreiber W, Fujimura S, Dale EA, Faustman DL (2003) Islet regeneration during the reversal of auto-immune diabetes in NOD mice. Science 302:1223–1227

25. Nagata H, Ito M, Shirota C, Edge A, McCowan TC, Fox IJ (2003) Route of hepatocyte delivery affects hepatocyte engraftment in the spleen. Transplantation 76:732–734

26. Kocher AA, Schuster MD, Szabolcs MJ, Takuma S, Burkhoff D, Wang J, Homma S, Edwards NM, Itescu S (2001) Neovascularization of ischemic myocardium by human bone-marrow-derived angioblasts prevents cardiomyocyte apoptosis, reduces remodeling and improves cardiac function. Nat Med 7:430–436

27. Penn MS, Francis GS, Ellis SG, Young JB, McCarthy PM, Topol EJ (2002) Autologous cell transplantation for the treatment of damaged myocardium. Prog Cardiovasc Dis 45:21–32

28. Peron JM, Couderc B, Rochaix P, Douin-Echinard V, Asnacios A, Souque A, Voigt JJ, Buscail L, Vinel JP, Favre G (2004) Treatment of murine hepatocellular carcinoma using genetically modified cells to express interleukin-12. J Gastroenterol Hepatol 19:388–396

29. Roth JA, Grammer SF (2004) Gene replacement therapy for non-small cell lung cancer: a review. Hematol Oncol Clin North Am 18:215–229

30. Liechty KW, MacKenzie TC, Shaaban AF, Radu A, Moseley AM, Deans R, Marshak DR, Flake AW (2000) Human mesenchymal stem cells engraft and demonstrate site-specific differentiation after in utero transplantation in sheep. Nat Med 6:1282–1286

31. Barron V, Lyons E, Stenson-Cox C, McHugh PE, Pandit A (2003) Bioreactors for cardiovascular cell and tissue growth: a review. Ann Biomed Eng 31:1017–1030

32. Dutt K, Harris-Hooker S, Ellerson DL, Kumar R, Hunt R (2003) Generation of 3D retina-like structures from a human retinal cell line in a NASA bioreactor. Cell Transplant 12:717–731

33. Vunjak-Novakovic G (2003) The fundamentals of tissue engineering: scaffolds and bioreactors. Novartis Found Symp 249:34–46

34. Hall CW, Liotta D, De Bakey ME (1966) Artificial skin. Trans Am Soc Artif Intern Organs 12:340–345

35. Wright KA, Nadire KB, Busto P, Tubo R, McPherson JM, Wentworth BM (1998) Alternative delivery of keratinocytes using a polyurethane membrane and the implications for its use in the treatment of full-thickness burn injury. Burns 24:7–17

36. Carsin H, Ainaud P, Le Bever H, Rives J, Lakhel A, Stephanazzi J, Lambert F, Perrot J (2000) Cultured epithelial autografts in extensive burn coverage of severely traumatized patients: a five year single-center experience with 30 patients. Burns 26:379–387

37. Eaglstein WH (1998) Dermagraft treatment of diabetic ulcers. J Dermatol 25:803–804

38. Marston WA, Hanft J, Norwood P, Pollak R, Group DDFUS (2003) The efficacy and safety of Dermagraft in improving the healing of chronic diabetic foot ulcers: results of a prospective randomized trial. Diabetes Care 26:1701–1705

39. Fivenson D, Scherschun L (2003) Clinical and economic impact of Apligraf for the treatment of nonhealing venous leg ulcers. Int J Dermatol 42:960–965

40. Bannasch H, Fohn M, Unterberg T, Bach AD, Weyand B, Stark GB (2003) Skin tissue engineering. Clin Plast Surg 30:573–579

41. Vacanti CA, Langer R, Schloo B, Vacanti JP (1991) Synthetic polymers seeded with chondrocytes provide a template for new cartilage formation. Plast Reconstr Surg 88:753–759

42. Kim WS, Vacanti JP, Cima L, Mooney D, Upton J, Puelacher WC, Vacanti CA (1994) Cartilage engineered in predetermined shapes employing cell transplantation on synthetic biodegradable polymers. Plast Reconstr Surg 94:233–237

43. Kim WS, Vacanti CA, Upton J, Vacanti JP (1994) Bone defect repair with tissue-engineered cartilage. Plast Reconstr Surg 94:580–584

44. Vacanti CA, Kim WS, Schloo B, Upton J, Vacanti JP (1994) Joint resurfacing with cartilage grown in situ from cell-polymer structures. Am J Sports Med 22:485–488

45. Brittberg M, Lindahl A, Nilsson A, Ohlsson C, Isaksson O, Peterson L (1994) Treatment of deep cartilage defects in the knee with autologous chondrocyte transplantation. N Engl J Med 331:889–895

46. Puelacher WC, Mooney D, Langer R, Upton J, Vacanti JP, Vacanti CA (1994) Design of nasoseptal cartilage replacements synthesized from biodegradable polymers and chondrocytes. Biomaterials 15:774–778

47. Puelacher WC, Wisser J, Vacanti CA, Ferraro NF, Jaramillo D, Vacanti JP (1994) Temporomandibular joint disc replacement made by tissue-engineered growth of cartilage. J Oral Maxillofac Surg 52:1172–1177

48. Vacanti CA, Cima LG, Ratkowski D, Upton J, Vacanti JP (1992) Tissue engineered growth of new cartilage in the shape of a human ear using synthetic polymers seeded with chondrocytes. Mater Res Soc Symp Proc 252:36–374

49. Cao Y, Vacanti JP, Paige KT, Upton J, Vacanti CA (1997) Transplantation of chondrocytes utilizing a polymer-cell construct to produce tissue-engineered cartilage in the shape of a human ear. Plast Reconstr Surg 100:297–302

50. Sakata J, Vacanti CA, Schloo B, Healy GB, Langer R, Vacanti JP (1994) Tracheal composites tissue engineered from chondrocytes, tracheal epithelial cells, and synthetic degradable scaffolding. Transplant Proc 26:2209–2210

51. Vacanti CA, Paige KT, Kim WS, Sakata J, Upton J, Vacanti JP (1994) Experimental tracheal replacement using tissue-engineered cartilage. J Pediatr Surg 29:201–204

52. Kojima K, Bonassar LJ, Roy AK, Vacanti CA, Cortiella J (2002) Autologous tissue-engineered trachea with sheep nasal chondrocytes. J Thorac Cardiovasc Surg 123:1177–1184

53. Kojima K, Bonassar LJ, Roy AK, Mizuno H, Cortiella J, Vacanti CA (2003) A composite tissue-engineered trachea using sheep nasal chondrocyte and epithelial cells. FASEB J 17:823–828

54. Kojima K, Bonassar LJ, Ignotz RA, Syed K, Cortiella J, Vacanti CA (2003) Comparison of tracheal and nasal chondrocytes for tissue engineering of the trachea. Ann Thorac Surg 76:1884–1888

55. Rotter N, Bonassar LJ, Tobias G, Lebl M, Roy AK, Vacanti CA (2001) Age dependence of cellular properties of human septal cartilage: implications for tissue engineering. Arch Otolaryngol Head Neck Surg 127:1248–1252

56. Fuchs JR, Terada S, Hannouche D, Ochoa ER, Vacanti JP, Fauza DO (2003) Engineered fetal cartilage: structural and functional analysis in vitro. J Pediatr Surg 37:1720–1725

57. Pei M, Solchaga LA, Seidel J, Zeng L, Vunjak-Novakovic G, Caplan AI, Freed LE (2002) Bioreactors mediate the effectiveness of tissue engineering scaffolds. FASEB J 16:1691–1694

58. Park S, Hung CT, Ateshian GA (2004) Mechanical response of bovine articular cartilage under dynamic unconfined compression loading at physiological stress levels. Osteoarthritis Cartilage 12:65–73

59. Fauza DO, Marler JJ, Koka R, Forse RA, Mayer JE, Vacanti JP (2001) Fetal tissue engineering: diaphragmatic replacement. J Pediatr Surg 36:146–151

60. Fuchs JR, Terada S, Ochoa ER, Vacanti JP, Fauza DO (2002) Fetal tissue engineering: in utero tracheal augmentation in an ovine model. J Pediatr Surg 37:1000–1006

61. Elisseeff J, Anseth K, Sims D, McIntosh W, Randolph M, Yaremchuk M, Langer R (1999) Transdermal photopolymerization of poly(ethylene oxide)-based injectable hydrogels for tissue-engineered cartilage. Plast Reconstr Surg 104:1014–1022

62. Nguyen KT, West JL (2002) Photopolymerizable hydrogels for tissue engineering applications. Biomaterials 23:4307–4314

63. Williams CG, Kim TK, Taboas A, Malik A, Manson P, Elisseeff J (2003) In vitro chondrogenesis of bone marrow-derived mesenchymal stem cells in a photopolymerizing hydrogel. Tissue Eng 9:679–688

64. Bauer TW, Togawa D (2003) Bone graft substitutes: towards a more perfect union. Orthopedics 26:925–926

65. Chapman MW, Bucholz R, Cornell C (1997) Treatment of acute fractures with a collagen-calcium phosphate graft material: a randomized clinical trial. J Bone Joint Surg Am 79:495–502

66. Irwin RB, Bernhard M, Biddinger A (2001) Coralline hydroxyapatite as bone substitute in orthopedic oncology. Am J Orthop 30:544–550

67. Buchholz RW (2002) Nonallograft osteoconductive bone graft substitutes. Clin Orthop 395:44–52

68. Puelacher WC, Vacanti JP, Ferraro NF, Schloo B, Vacanti CA (1996) Femoral shaft reconstruction using tissue-engineered growth of bone. Int J Oral Maxillofac Surg 25:223–228

69. Isogai N, Landis WJ, Kim TH, Gerstenfeld LC, Upton J, Vacanti JP (1999) Formation of phalanges and small joints by tissue-engineering. J Bone Joint Surg Am 81:306–316

70. Isogai N, Landis WJ, Mori R, Gotoh Y, Gerstenfeld LC, Upton J, Vacanti JP (2000) Experimental use of fibrin glue to induce site-directed osteogenesis from cultured periosteal cells. Plast Reconstr Surg 105:953–963

71. Vacanti CA, Bonassar LJ, Vacanti MP, Shufflebarger J (2001) Replacement of an avulsed phalanx with tissue-engineered bone. N Engl J Med 344:1511–1514

72. Caplan AI (1991) Mesenchymal stem cells. J Orthop Res 8:641–650

73. Bruder SP, Fink DJ, Caplan AI (1994) Mesenchymal stem cells in bone development, bone repair, and skeletal regeneration therapy. J Cell Biochem 56:283–294

74. Pittenger MF, Mackay AM, Beck SC, Jaiswal RK, Douglas R, Mosca JD, Moorman MA, Simonetti DW, Craig S, Marshak DR (1999) Multilineage potential of adult human mesenchymal stem cells. Science 284:143–147

75. Ishaug SL, Crane GM, Miller MJ, Yasko AW, Yazemski MJ, Mikos AG (1997) Bone formation by three-dimensional stromal osteoblast culture in biodegradable polymer scaffolds. J Biomed Mater Res 36:17–28

76. Goldstein AS, Zhu G, Morris GE, Meslenyi RK, Mikos AG (1999) Effect of osteoblastic culture conditions on the structure of poly(dl-lactic-co-glycolic acid) foam scaffolds. Tissue Eng 5:421–433

77. Terai H, Hannouche D, Ochoa E, Yamano Y, Vacanti JP (2002) In vitro engineering of bone using a rotational oxygen-permeable bioreactor system. Mat Sci Eng C 20:3–8

78. Abukawa H, Terai H, Hannouche D, Vacanti JP, Kaban LB, Troulis MJ (2003) Formation of a mandibular condyle in vitro by tissue engineering. J Oral Maxillofac Surg 61:94–100

79. Nakagawa K, Abukawa H, Shin M, Terai H, Troulis MJ, Vacanti JP (2004) Osteoclastogenesis on tissue-engineered bone. Tissue Eng 10:93–100

80. Zeltinger J, Sherwood JK, Graham DA, Mueller R, Griffith LG (2001) Effect of pore size and void fraction on cellular adhesion, proliferation, and matrix deposition. Tissue Eng 7:557–572

81. Yoshimoto H, Shin M, Vacanti JP (2003) A biodegradable nanofiber scaffold by electrospinning and its potential for bone tissue engineering. Biomaterials 24:2077–2082

82. Koegler WS, Griffith LG (2004) Osteoblast response to PLGA tissue engineering scaffolds with PEO modified surface chemistries and demonstration of patterned cell response. Biomaterials 15:2819–2830

83. Lin CY, Kikuchi N, Hollister SJ (2004) A novel method for biomaterial scaffold internal architecture design to match bone elastic properties with desired porosity. J Biomech 37:623–636

84. Sikavitsas VI, Bancroft GN, Holtorf HL, Jansen JA, Mikos AG (2003) Mineralized matrix deposition by marrow stromal osteoblasts in 3D perfusion culture increases with increasing fluid shear forces. Proc Natl Acad Sci USA 100:14683–14688

85. Meinel L, Karageorgiou V, Fajardo R, Snyder B, Shinde-Patil V, Zichner L, Kaplan D, Langer R, Vunjak-Novakovic G (2004) Bone tissue engineering using human mesenchymal stem cells: effects of scaffold material and medium flow. Ann Biomed Eng 32:112–122

86. Caplan AI (2000) Mesenchymal stem cells and gene therapy. Clin Orthop 379:S67–S70

87. Chamberlain JR, Schwarze U, Wang PR, Hirata RK, Hankenson KD, Pace JM, Underwood RA, Song KM, Sussman M, Byers PH, Russell DW (2004) Gene targeting in stem cells from individuals with osteogenesis imperfecta. Science 303:1198–1201

88. Thompson JS, Iyer KR, DiBaise JK, Young RL, Brown CR, Langnas AN (2003) Short bowel syndrome and Crohn's disease. J Gastrointest Surg 7:1069–1072

89. Kaufman SS, Gondolesi GE, Fishbein TM (2003) Parenteral nutrition associated liver disease. Semin Neonatol 8:375–381

90. Vernon AH, Georgeson KE (2001) Surgical options for short bowel syndrome. Semin Pediatr Surg 10:91–98

91. Carlson GL (2003) Surgical management of intestinal failure. Proc Nutr Soc 62:711–718

92. Mittal NK, Tzakis AG, Kato T, Thompson JF (2003) Current status of small bowel transplantation in children: update 2003. Pediatr Clin North Am 50:1419–1433

93. Organ GM, Mooney DJ, Hansen LK, Schloo B, Vacanti JP (1992) Transplantation of enterocytes utilizing polymer-cell constructs to produce a neointestine. Transplant Proc 24:3009–3011

94. Organ GM, Mooney DJ, Hansen LK, Schloo B, Vacanti JP (1993) Enterocyte transplantation using cell-polymer devices to create intestinal epithelial-lined tubes. Transplant Proc 25:998–1001

95. Choi RS, Vacanti JP (1997) Preliminary studies of tissue-engineered intestine using isolated epithelial organoid units on tubular synthetic biodegradable scaffolds. Transplant Proc 29:848–851

96 Choi RS, Riegler M, Pothoulakis C, Kim BS, Mooney D, Vacanti M, Vacanti JP (1998) Studies of brush border enzymes, basement membrane components, and electrophysiology of tissue-engineered neointestine. J Pediatr Surg 33:991–996

97. Kim SS, Kaihara S, Benvenuto MS, Choi RS, Kim BS, Mooney DJ, Taylor GA, Vacanti JP (1999) Regenerative signals for intestinal epithelial organoid units transplanted on biodegradable polymer scaffolds for tissue engineering of small intestine. Transplantation 672:227–233

98. Kim SS, Kaihara S, Benvenuto MS, Choi RS, Kim BS, Mooney DJ, Taylor GA, Vacanti JP (1999) Regenerative signals for tissue-engineered small intestine. Transplant Proc 31:657–670

99. Kaihara S, Kim SS, Benvenuto M, Choi RS, Kim BS, Mooney D, Tanaka K, Vacanti JP (1999) Successful anastomosis between tissue-engineered intestine and native small bowel. Transplantation 67:241–245

100. Kaihara S, Kim SS, Benvenuto M, Choi RS, Kim BS, Mooney D, Tanaka K, Vacanti JP (1999) Anastomosis between tissue-engineered intestine and native small bowel. Transplant Proc 31:661–662

101. Kaihara S, Kim SS, Benvenuto M, Choi RS, Kim BS, Mooney D, Tanaka K, Vacanti JP (1999) End-to-end anastomosis between tissue-engineered intestine and native small bowel. Tissue Eng 5:339–346

102. Kim SS, Kaihara S, Benvenuto MS, Choi RS, Kim BS, Mooney DJ, Vacanti JP (1999) Effects of anastomosis of tissue-engineered neointestine to native small bowel. J Surg Res 87:6–13

103. Kaihara S, Kim SS, Kim BS, Mooney DJ, Tanaka K, Vacanti JP (2000) Long-term follow-up of tissue-engineered intestine after anastomosis to native small bowel. Transplantation 69:1927–1932

104. Grikscheit TC, Ogilvie JB, Ochoa ER, Alsberg E, Mooney D, Vacanti JP (2003) Tissue-engineered colon exhibits function in vivo. Surgery 132:200–204

105. Grikscheit TC, Ochoa ER, Ramsanahie A, Alsberg E, Mooney D, Whang EE, Vacanti JP (2003) Tissue-engineered large intestine resembles native colon with appropriate in vitro physiology and architecture. Ann Surg 238:35–41

106. Grikscheit TC, Srinivasan A, Vacanti JP (2003) Tissue-engineered stomach: a preliminary report of a versatile in vivo model with therapeutic potential. J Pediatr Surg 38:1305–1309

107. Maemura T, Shin M, Sato M, Mochizuki H, Vacanti JP (2003) A tissue-engineered stomach as a replacement of the native stomach. Transplantation 576:61–65

108. Gardner-Thorpe J, Grikscheit TC, Ito H, Perez A, Ashley SW, Vacanti JP, Whang EE (2003) Angiogenesis in tissue-engineered small intestine. Tissue Eng 9:1255–1261

109. Lamm P, Juchem G, Milz S, Schuffenhauer M, Reichart B (2001) Autologous endothelialized vein allograft: a solution in the search for small-caliber grafts in coronary artery bypass graft operations. Circulation 104:I108–I114

110. Bos GW, Poot AA, Beugeling T, van Aken WG, Feijen J (1998) Small-diameter vascular graft prostheses: current status. Arch Physiol Biochem 106:100–115

111. Miwa H, Matsuda T (1994) An integrated approach to the design and engineering of hybrid arterial prostheses. J Vasc Surg 19:658–667

112. Weinberg CB, Bell E (1986) A blood vessel model constructed from collagen and cultured vascular cells. Science 231:397–400

113. L'Heureux N, Paquet S, Labbe R, Germain L, Auger FA (1998) A completely biological tissue-engineered human blood vessel. FASEB J 12:47–56

114. Huynh T, Abraham G, Murray J, Brockbank K, Hagen PO, Sullivan S (1999) Remodeling of an acellular collagen graft into a physiologically responsive neovessel. Nat Biotechnol 17:1083–1086

115. Niklason LE, Gao J, Abbott WM, Hirschi KK, Houser S, Marini R, Langer R (1999) Functional arteries grown in vitro. Science 284:489–493

116. Shinoka T, Shum-Tim D, Ma PX, Tanel RE, Isogai N, Langer R, Vacanti JP, Mayer JEJ (1998) Creation of viable pulmonary artery autografts through tissue engineering. J Thorac Cardiovasc Surg 115:536–545

117. Stock UA, Sakamoto T, Hatsuoka S, Martin DP, Nagashima M, Moran AM, Moses MA, Khalil PN, Schoen FJ, Vacanti JP, Mayer JEJ (2000) Patch augmentation of the pulmonary artery with bioabsorbable polymers and autologous cell seeding. J Thorac Cardiovasc Surg 120:1158–1167

118. Watanabe M, Shin'oka T, Tohyama S, Hibino N, Konuma T, Matsumura G, Kosaka Y, Ishida T, Imai Y, Yamakawa M, Ikada Y, Morita S (2001) Tissue-engineered vascular autograft: inferior vena cava replacement in a dog model. Tissue Eng 74:429–439

119. Shin'oka T, Imai Y, Ikada Y (2001) Transplantation of a tissue-engineered pulmonary artery. N Engl J Med 344:532–533

120. Naito Y, Imai Y, Shin'oka T, Kashiwagi J, Aoki M, Watanabe M, Matsumura G, Kosaka Y, Konuma T, Hibino N, Murata A, Miyake T, Kurosawa H (2003) Successful clinical application of tissue-engineered graft for extracardiac Fontan operation. J Thorac Cardiovasc Surg 125:129–130

121. Matsumura G, Hibino N, Ikada Y, Kurosawa H, Shin'oka T (2003) Successful application of tissue engineered vascular autografts: clinical experience. Biomaterials 24:2303–2308

122. Matsumura G, Miyagawa-Tomita S, Shin'oka T, Ikada Y, Kurosawa H (2003) First evidence that bone marrow cells contribute to the construction of tissue-engineered vascular autografts in vivo. Circulation 108:1729–1734

123. Isomatsu Y, Shinoka T, Matsumura G, Hibino N, Konuma T, Nagatsu M, Kurosawa H (2003) Extracardiac total cavopulmonary connection using a tissue-engineered graft. J Thorac Cardiovasc Surg 126:1958–1962

124. American Liver Foundation (2005) Annual report, 2005. American Liver Foundation, Cedar Grove, N.J.

125. Starzl TE, Tzakis A, Fung JJ, Todo S, Demetris AJ, Manez R, Marino IR, Valdivia L, Murase N (1994) Prospects of clinical xenotransplantation. Transplant Proc 26:1082–1088

126. Schmidt HH, Tietge UJ, Manns MP (1997) Perspectives of liver cell transplantation: a review. Hepatogastroenterology 44:1013–1018

127. Busuttil RW, Goss JA (1999) Split liver transplantation. Ann Surg 229:313–321

128. Kilic M, Seu P, Stribling RJ, Ghalib R, Goss JA (2001) In situ splitting of the cadaveric liver for two adult recipients. Transplantation 72:1853–1858

129. Kasahara M, Uryuhara K, Kaihara S, Kozaki K, Fujimoto Y, Ogura Y, Ogawa K, Oike F, Ueda M, Egawa H, Tanaka K (2003) Monosegmental living donor liver transplantation. Transplant Proc 35:1425–1426

130. Takada Y, Tanaka K (2004) Living related liver transplantation. Transplant Proc 36:271S–273S

131. Jaffe V, Darby H, Selden C, Hodgson HJ (1988) The growth of transplanted liver cells within the pancreas. Transplantation 45:497–498

132. Gupta S, Aragona E, Vemuru RP, Bhargava KK, Burk RD, Chowdhury JR (1991) Permanent engraftment and function of hepatocytes delivered to the liver: implications for gene therapy and liver repopulation. Hepatology 14:144–149

133. Kusano M, Sawa M, Jiang B, Kino S, Itoh K, Sakata H, Katoh K, Mito M (1992) Proliferation and differentiation of fetal liver cells transplanted into rat spleen. Transplant Proc 24:2960–2961

134. Demetriou AA, Whiting JF, Feldman D, Levenson SM, Chowdhury NR, Moscioni AD, Kram M, Chowdhury JR (1986) Replacement of liver function in rats by transplantation of microcarrier-attached hepatocytes. Science 223:1190–1192

135. Dixit V, Darvasi R, Arthur M, Lewin K, Gitnick G (1993) Cryopreserved microencapsulated hepatocytes--transplantation studies in Gunn rats. Transplantation 55:616–622

136. Vacanti JP, Morse MA, Saltzman WM, Domb AJ, Perez-Atayde A, Langer R (1988) Selective cell transplantation using bioabsorbable artificial polymers as matrices. J Pediatr Surg 23:3–9

137. Johnson LB, Aiken J, Mooney D, Schloo BL, Griffith-Cima L, Langer R, Vacanti JP (1994) The mesentery as a laminated vascular bed for hepatocyte transplantation. Cell Transplant 3:273–281

138. Fontaine M, Schloo B, Jenkins R, Uyama S, Hansen L, Vacanti JP (1995) Human hepatocyte isolation and transplantation into an athymic rat, using prevascularized cell polymer constructs. J Pediatr Surg 30:56–60

139. Wake MC, Mikos AG, Sarakinos G, Vacanti JP, Langer R (1995) Dynamics of fibrovascular tissue ingrowth in hydrogel foams. Cell Transplant 4:275–279

140. Kaufmann PM, Sano K, Uyama S, Schloo B, Vacanti JP (1994) Heterotopic hepatocyte transplantation using three-dimensional polymers: evaluation of the stimulatory effects by portacaval shunt or islet cell cotransplantation. Transplant Proc 26:3343–3345

141. Kaufmann PM, Sano K, Uyama S, Takeda T, Vacanti JP (1994) Heterotopic hepatocyte transplantation: assessing the impact of hepatotrophic stimulation. Transplant Proc 26:2240–2241

142. Mooney DJ, Kaufmann PM, Sano K, McNamara KM, Vacanti JP, Langer R (1994) Transplantation of hepatocytes using porous, biodegradable sponges. Transplant Proc 26:3425–3426

143. Sano K, Cusick RA, Lee H, Pollok JM, Kaufmann PM, Uyama S, Mooney D, Langer R, Vacanti JP (1996) Regenerative signals for heterotopic hepatocyte transplantation. Transplant Proc 28:1857–1858

144. Asonuma K, Gilbert JC, Stein JE, Takeda T, Vacanti JP (1992) Quantitation of transplanted hepatic mass necessary to cure the Gunn rat model of hyperbilirubinemia. Transplant Proc 27:298–301

145. Uyama S, Kaufmann PM, Takeda T, Vacanti JP (1993) Delivery of whole liver-equivalent hepatocyte mass using polymer devices and hepatotrophic stimulation. Transplantation 55:932–935

146. Takeda T, Kim TH, Lee SK, Langer R, Vacanti JP (1995) Hepatocyte transplantation in biodegradable polymer scaffolds using the Dalmatian dog model of hyperuricosuria. Transplant Proc 27:635–636

147. Takeda T, Murphy S, Uyama S, Organ GM, Schloo BL, Vacanti JP (1995) Hepatocyte transplantation in swine using prevascularized polyvinyl alcohol sponges. Tissue Eng 1:253–262

148. Takeda T, Vacanti JP (1995) Hepatocyte transplantation in the Dalmatian dog model of hyperuricosuria. Tissue Engineering. Tissue Eng 1:355–360

149. Lee H, Cusick RA, Browne F, Ho Kim T, Ma PX, Utsunomiya H, Langer R, Vacanti JP (2002) Local delivery of basic fibroblast growth factor increases both angiogenesis and engraftment of hepatocytes in tissue-engineered polymer devices. Transplantation 73:1589–1593

150. Mikos AG, Bao Y, Cima LG, Ingber DE, Vacanti JP, Langer R (1993) Preparation of poly(glycolic acid) bonded fiber structures for cell attachment and transplantation. J Biomed Mater Res 27:183–189

151. Kaihara S, Kim S, Kim BS, Mooney DJ, Tanaka K, Vacanti JP (2000) Survival and function of rat hepatocytes cocultured with nonparenchymal cells or sinusoidal endothelial cells on biodegradable polymers under flow conditions. J Pediatr Surg 35:1287–1290

152. Kim SS, Sundback CA, Kaihara S, Benvenuto MS, Kim BS, Mooney DJ, Vacanti JP (2000) Dynamic seeding and in vitro culture of hepatocytes in a flow perfusion system. Tissue Eng 6:39–44

153. Sachs EM, Cima MJ, Williams P, Brancazio D, Cornie J (1992) Three dimensional printing. J Eng Ind 114:481–488

154. Griffith LG, Wu B, Cima MJ, Powers MJ, Chaignaud B, Vacanti JP (1997) In vitro organogenesis of liver tissue. Ann NY Acad Sci 831:382–397

155. Kim SS, Utsunomiya H, Koski JA, Wu BM, Cima MJ, Sohn J, Mukai K, Griffith LG, Vacanti JP (1998) Survival and function of hepatocytes on a novel three-dimensional synthetic biodegradable polymer scaffold with an intrinsic network of channels. Ann Surg 228:8–13

156. Madou M (2002) Fundamentals of microfabrication: the science of miniaturization, 2nd edn. CRC, Boca Raton, Flal.

157. Kaihara S, Borenstein J, Koka R, Lalan S, Ochoa ER, Ravens M, Pien H, Cunningham B, Vacanti JP (2000) Silicon micromachining to tissue engineer branched vascular channels for liver fabrication. Tissue Eng 6:105–117

158. Kaazempur-Mofrad MR, Vacanti JP, Kamm RD (2001) Computational modeling of blood flow and rheology in fractal microvascular networks. Comp Fluid Solid Mech 2:864–867

159. Shin M, Matsuda K, Ishii O, Terai H, Kaazempur-Mofrad M, Borenstein J, Detmar M, Vacanti JP (2002) Microvascular networks for tissue-engineered organs. 5th International Meeting of the Tissue Engineering Society International, Kobe, Japan

160. TIME (2000) The hottest jobs of the future. 22 May 2000

161. Lavine M, Roberts L, Smith O (2002) The bionic human. Science 295:995

162. Lysaght MJ, Hazlehurst AL (2004) Tissue engineering: the end of the beginning. Tissue Eng 10:309–320

163. Koike N, Fukumura D, Gralla O, Au P, Schechner JS, Jain RK (2004) Tissue engineering: creation of long-lasting blood vessels. Nature 428:138–139

164. LeGeros RZ (2002) Properties of osteoconductive biomaterials: calcium phosphates. Clin Orthop 395:81–98

165. Lickorish D, Ramshaw JA, Werkmeister JA, Glattauer V, Howlett CR (2004) Collagen-hydroxyapatite composite prepared by biomimetic process. J Biomed Mater Res 68A:19–27

166. Oral E, Peppas NA (2004) Responsive and recognitive hydrogels using star polymers. J Biomed Mater Res 68A:439–447

167. Tabata Y, Miyao M, Yamamoto M, Ikada Y (1999) Vascularization into a porous sponge by sustained release of basic fibroblast growth factor. J Biomater Sci Polym Ed 10:957–968

168. Smith MK, Peters MC, Richardson TP, Garbern JC, Mooney DJ (2004) Locally enhanced angiogenesis promotes transplanted cell survival. Tissue Eng 10:63–71

169. Shimizu T, Yamato M, Isoi Y, Akutsu T, Setomaru T, Abe K, Kikuchi A, Umezu M, Okano T (2002) Fabrication of pulsatile cardiac tissue grafts using a novel 3-dimensional cell sheet manipulation technique and temperature responsive cell culture surfaces. Circ Res 90:e40

170. Hartgerink JD, Beniash E, Stupp SI (2001) Self-assembly and mineralization of peptide-amphiphile nanofibers. Science 294:1684–1688

171. Zhang S (2003) Fabrication of novel biomaterials through molecular self-assembly. Nat Biotechnol 21:1171–1178

172. Pratt AB, Weber FE, Schmoekel HG, Muller R, Hubbell JA (2004) Synthetic extracellular matrices for in situ tissue engineering. Biotechnol Bioeng 86:27–36

173. Atala A (2004) Tissue engineering for the replacement of organ function in the genitourinary system. Am J Transplant 4:58–73

Part VI
Beyond the Future

Adapting to Future Technologies

17

Richard M. Satava*

Advanced technologies disrupt the very way that surgery will be performed in the future. There will also be a fundamental change in how medicine and scientific research will be conducted, beyond the hallowed scientific method. There will be many different new surgical approaches, from non-invasive to biosurgery, with different robotic and autonomous systems that will require new skills and new training methods. Surgical education will become criterion-based and life long, with continuous assessment.

17.1 Introduction

There has never been such an accelerated discovery of new technologies as during the past century; even the Renaissance pales in comparison. In addition, the dissemination of these technologies, facilitated by the developing transportation and communication systems, has resulted in innovation becoming rapidly pervasive on a global scale. This is a self-accelerating process: As new concepts and ideas are quickly disseminated throughout the world, researchers anywhere have immediate access to the information that will rapidly drive their research to the next discovery. Amid this whirlwind of activity, the surgeon is being asked to provide careful and thoughtful clinical practice—to stay up to date and bring the latest technology to bear, while ensuring rigorous evaluation and resisting the temptation to jump on the bandwagon of the latest new discovery. This dichotomy will continue: rapid acceptance and application versus prolonged stringent evaluation. The following is an attempt to clarify the future trends so the practicing surgeon can adapt to change, and navigate between these two opposite poles.

17.2 The Scientific Method

Nothing is closer to the core of surgery than the principles of the scientific method by which we discover, evaluate, validate, and implement a new technology. Until the turn of the 20th century, surgery was guided by tradition. It was Nicholas Senn's seminal article in 1908, which pointed out that rather than tradition, a surgeon should rely upon experience [1]. No longer was it acceptable to continue the practices of old simply because it had become the custom; rather, Senn declared that surgeons should look at the experience and results of previous treatments and be guided by logical judgment in surgical practice. From this modest beginning, surgery evolved into the scientific method as we know it today: hypothesis, research, conclusion, and implementation. Laboratory research began to ascend and along with it came clinical trials. Studies were carefully designed and crafted, and then rigorously conducted to gather the evidence necessary to prove or disprove the hypothesis, and culminated in publication of the scientific evidence, which resulted in the acceptance by the surgical community at large. While this method has brought clarity and understanding out of chaos, the rigorous nature of the investigation has resulted in an extremely long time from discovery to validation to implementation. Often new technologies were invoked before the evidence was confirmed, much to the detriment of the patients (laparoscopic cholecystectomy with initial increased incidence of bile duct injuries, or various chemotherapeutic agents with either unintended side effects or lack of efficacy). The converse was also true; prolonged evaluation resulted in many patients not receiving life-saving therapy while awaiting the results of trials, or new surgical procedures not being implemented for decades until the completion of trials (such as laparoscopic colectomy). While it is not the intent to suggest that the current rigorous process is neither valid nor necessary, there is a method that has been implemented by the scientific community that has not been considered by the medical profession, modeling and simulation. There is some early implementation of simulation technologies being explored for rapid rational drug design and for understanding gene-based therapies. Sophisticated computer programs are being used to simulate the effects of literally millions of pos-

---

* The opinions or assertions contained herein are the private views of the authors and are not to be construed as official, or as reflecting the views of the Department of the Army, Department of the Navy, the Advanced Research Projects Agency, or the Department of Defense.

sible compounds, looking for the desired combinations and possible mechanisms of action. These simulations include the composition, structure, folding, bonding, etc., iterated over thousands of potential combinations to discover the most likely candidates for production and study. Thus a nearly infinite number of potential biochemical molecules are reduced to specific drugs or genetic sequences that are targeted and used in clinical trails. There is a primordial effort to take the next step, to test these candidate therapies through simulation on a "virtual cell" (in silico, or computational biology), before implementing them in clinical trials on patients. Following this example to its ultimate conclusion, it is anticipated that it will be possible to simulate an entire organ, or even a single patient or population of individuals, to test and evaluate drug or genetic therapy before implementing on patients. Perhaps all therapies—drugs, procedures, energy-directed therapy—will be simulated until validated before using on patients: in essence, a virtual clinical trial on millions of computer-simulated patients over 50 years completed in 1 week of computation on a computer. This will be a "predictive process of simulation", the ultimate clinical trial. Although it will take decades to improve the methodology, first principles already valid in engineering and other scientific disciplines demonstrate the significance of this methodology, especially in rapidly assessing a new technology. The result is a new way of technology application: discovery, laboratory investigation (scientific method), predictive simulation, clinical trial. In the near term, the use of the predictive simulation will be able to dramatically reduce the length and number of subjects required to demonstrate efficacy in clinical trials (as extrapolated by the use of simulation in industry). The ultimate goal is the removal of patients from clinical trials, just as there is now a transition of using simulation in surgical skills to decrease or eliminate the need of animals in training and assessment of surgeon competency.

With this new methodology the clinical surgeon must adapt to the changing basis of providing evidence. Clearly it is no longer acceptable to base treatment upon tradition without supporting evidence (evidence-based surgery). It will be prudent to watch the emerging evidence on the predictability of simulations, for only with carefully designed computer programming will the simulation actually match the predictability of clinical trials. What the new simulation technology will be able provide that clinical trials cannot is predictability in compressed time: days instead of decades. Thus, in reading manuscripts for the latest new technology, it is critical to look at the evidence for validity. While there are well-known statistical methods that are used as the benchmarks for validation today, the practicing surgeon may soon need to learn new benchmarks that prove the validity of a simulated clinical trial.

17.3   Interdisciplinary Medicine

As indicated above, we are just beginning to understand the extraordinary complexity of our world. Many of the new advances in technology have been due to the work of the interdisciplinary team, which has much greater knowledge than does any single investigator. Such a team could be composed of as few as two scientific fields, such as engineering and computer science for a new surgical instrument, or a large complex organization of computational mathematicians, engineers, biochemists, molecular biologists, statisticians, and clinical practitioners, such as the team approach for research in artificial organs. This also extends to the operating room, where surgical procedures are attaining a complexity that requires a team approach of anesthesiologist, surgeon, nurse, technician, etc., although new research in robotics may soon integrate the functions of the entire team into a single robotic system of surgeon, assistant surgeon, scrub nurse, and circulating nurse, all controlled by the surgeon at a surgical console outside the operating room without people. There may also be the sharing of responsibility when performing a procedure; for example, in vascular stenting of carotid arteries, should it be the surgeon, interventional radiologist, cardiologist, or a team composed of all three?

The challenge will be to craft strong, interdisciplinary teams. For the researcher it will be of colleagues in other major fields of science, and for the clinician it will be forging and training a smoothly functioning interdisciplinary team in the operating room, clinic, or office.

17.4   Multiaccess Surgery

Gone are the days of a surgical therapy with a single surgical approach: open surgery. Today many diseases may be treated by any number of procedures. For example, esophageal tumors can be treated by open surgical resection, minimally access (laparoscopic) surgery, image-guided ablation (cryo-, thermal-, radiofrequency), noninvasive destruction (transcutaneous high-intensity focused ultrasound, or HIFU), endovascular embolization, or by endoluminal (endoscopic) ablation and/or stenting. A number of diseases are best treated by dual or multiple modalities—combinations of minimally invasive and hand-assisted, endoluminal, laparoscopic, and so on. Such approaches, usually reserved for complicated diseases, will also require a preoperative planning session, using three-dimensional virtual reconstruction of the patient-specific anatomy from CT, MRI, or other modalities. While the results using such a preplanning process have unequivocally shown increase precision and decrease operative time for liver [3], plastic, craniofacial [4], neurosurgery, and other procedures, there is significant time devoted to the preoperative planning and rehearsal process for which there is currently no reimbursement. Eventually such a process will become routine for most complicated surgical cases; however, it is uncertain whether all procedures will be either planned or rehearsed ahead of time.

The busy practicing surgeon must strive to keep abreast of the new competing technologies and become trained and facile with as many approaches as is reasonable. An awareness of this multiple access trend must be monitored, for it may well impact, through regulation, how surgical practice may be conducted. It is conceivable that decades from now, surgeons will be required to rehearse all surgical procedures on the patient's three-dimensional reconstructed anatomy before being allowed to operate on that patient.

17.5   Information Technologies

The ubiquitous access in a timely fashion to critical information is changing the daily practice of surgery on very simple but many crucial levels. Knowledge about a patient and all his or her tests was kept in the chart at the bedside or in the memory of the surgeon. Today that information resides on a central server, accessible anytime and anywhere through computer stations in the hospital, clinic, or office, or instantly at the bedside or parking lot using personal digital assistants (PDAs) or other communication devices. In addition, knowledge about a particular disease or the latest clinical trial results were previously contained in journals in the library or surgeon's office; that information is also available immediately through a computer or PDA. Likewise, with new wireless sensors attached to patients, vital signs will be made available on the server anytime from anywhere. The result is that the surgeon knows a great deal about the practice of medicine and their specific patients, in real time. The challenge will be trying to sort out the most important information and apply the decision making for the best outcomes.

Information systems are also becoming enterprises, supporting the entire hospital system for the patient and for efficient hospital management. There is a trend to patient-centric medicine: focusing all the information around a single patient's record, rather than focusing each functional piece of information (X-ray, laboratory test, etc.) in different departments. In addition a longitudinal record, from moment of entry into the hospital system until beyond final discharge, the entire patient encounter will be documented, tracked, billed, and analyzed for outcomes: clinical, administrative

and financial. The University of Maryland has an innovative, integrated perioperative system, which tracks the patient from admission to outpatient surgery until discharge later that day, including the full surgical procedure [5]. Sophisticated vision recognition systems combined with smart tags monitor the patient, operating team, and operating theater and, supported by intelligent software and inference engines, automatically deduce and document the patient's progress from preoperative to postoperative care. Tracking personnel reduces lost time, trying to bring the operating team together in a timely fashion, while electronically labeling equipment and supplies permits just-in-time inventory and supply chain management.

The amount of authority the surgeon will be able to retain continues to diminish, especially in a time when automated information systems can much more efficiently perform processes and report outcomes than humans. As a busy clinical surgeon strives to spend more time seeing more patients and performing more surgical procedures, the administrative requirements and bureaucratic burdens dramatically decrease efficiency. The surgeon must adapt, and the most efficient way is to learn and harness the new technologies, rather that abdicating authority to administrators or becoming a slave to the technology.

17.6   Surgical Education and Certification

The paradigm shift in surgical education is from time-based training (e.g., 5 years of surgical residency, and then graduate with a subjective agreement by experts of the surgeon's basic training) to the new objective, criterion-, or proficiency-based training. The earlier model of mentoring (supplemented by knowledge acquisition and testing: lectures followed by written tests) resulted in a subjective assessment of performance, especially of technical procedural skills. The 1980s and 1990s saw the emergence of clinical problem-based learning, standardized patients for the Objective Structured Clinical Exam (OSCE), and the Objective Structured Assessment of Technical Skills (OSATS) [6] and McGill Inanimate System for Training and Evaluation of Laparoscopic Skills (MISTELS) [7]. Along with the recent validation studies on virtual reality surgical simulators such as the Minimally Invasive Surgical Training – Virtual Reality (MIST-VR) [8], a new benchmark in surgical training has been set: objective assessment based upon expert-derived criterion for proficiency. This is the paradigm shift. Following the lead of the Royal Colleges of Surgeons in establishing standardized curriculum in basic skills in training and evaluation, the American Council of Graduate Medical Education and the American Board of Medical Specialties in the United States have added the dimension of an increased rigor by defining the components of competency to be achieved through such structured curricula with objective performance metrics. Although still in transition, the training of a surgeon is on a path of objectively documented acquisition of skills to a predefined level of proficiency in formal laboratory setting (rather than on patients), complimented with continuous evaluation during training and throughout the clinical career.

To the practicing surgeon, the phrase *life-long learning* takes on greater significance—no longer is it exclusively a professional obligation internalized in every surgeon when the Hippocratic Oath is taken; it is now a regulation that will be continuously monitored and evaluated. It is necessary to adapt to this new environment of mandatory training for any (new) procedures, of continuous learning with assessment, and of auditing surgical practice performance for acceptable outcomes. Failure to adapt will result in loss of surgical practice privileges.

17.7 Surgical Simulation

Surgical simulation deserves a separate emphasis because it has a larger role than only in surgical education. Unquestionably, surgical simulation will continue to grow, developing newer, more sophisticated skills trainers that more closely approximate reality and that address abilities beyond basic skills such as simulating entire procedures. However, it must be kept in mind that a simulator is simply a tool—albeit a powerful tool—to supplement a total educational curriculum. It is essential to incorporate the didactic teaching of anatomy, steps of a procedure, and potential errors, along with expected outcomes of skills training and embed these into a curriculum that includes the simulator. Continuous feedback while training (an automatic function of any proper simulator) provides the methodology for a goal-oriented, criterion-based curriculum that permits the student to learn at his or her own pace, on his or her own time, and with automatic mentoring. In addition, an over-arching curriculum must be developed for each residency training year that describes all the surgical procedures for which the resident must obtain proficiency. No longer will it be acceptable to have exposure only to those diseases and surgical procedures that happen to occur when the resident is on a clinical rotation; it will be necessary to agree upon a fundamental curriculum of all the important procedures a resident must learn (and become proficient) and provide simulations of all these possibilities (a digital library of procedures) so every resident will perform to criterion each important surgical procedure before

graduating—a very large challenge that will last decades to achieve. This same methodology will become the standard for experienced surgeons who wish to adopt a new surgical procedure in their practice. No longer will it be acceptable to take a weekend course and return to operate on patients; rather, a longer period of training to proficiency followed by a period of mentoring and/or proctoring will be required.

Simulation is also being used for preoperative planning and then surgical rehearsal of complicated surgical procedures. Some of these difficult cases can be included in the digital library to train future surgeons as well. A unique opportunity arises with surgical robotics: The same surgical console that is used to perform an operation can be used to do preoperative planning, surgical rehearsal of a specific patient, or for education and training. The robotic system can keep track of hand motions and continuously assess performance, whether for the assessment of skills or documentation of proficiency, both during residency training and throughout clinical practice career. Thus the surgical robot has a role well beyond enhancement of surgical performance; it can incorporate training and assessment as an integral part of daily practice and life-long learning.

Until surgical robotic systems become ubiquitous, separate systems for training, assessment, planning, and rehearsal will need to be used. The practicing clinician should foster the use of robotics with inclusion of simulation capabilities. As technology both advances in sophistication and also incorporates the above simulation capabilities, surgeons should adapt by seizing the opportunity to train on simulators as well as preplan and rehearse their more difficult elective surgical cases.

17.8 Artificial Organs and Transplantation

Tissue engineering is making substantial progress [9] in growing synthetic organs, and transplantation is becoming successful in using less toxic immunosuppression, xenotransplantation, or other techniques. The result will be sufficient tissues and organs for transplantation, whether by modifying current techniques or through the use of various forms of tissue and genetic engineering. Once the need for artificial organs to substitute for organ failure has been satisfied, consideration can be made to the use of artificial organs for virtually any or every procedure. Today, surgeons practice organ conservation; however, with an adequate supply of artificial organs, surgeons may train to proficiency in one operation per organ system: remove and replace the entire organ in most every circumstance. There will be no need for dozens of different procedures in the surgeon's armamentarium, rather, one procedure per organ. It may be conceivable that some day, rather than repair organs, surgeons will simply remove and replace any diseased organ, just as automobile parts are no longer repaired, but simply replaced by a new and better part.

17.9 Surgical Systems and Robotics

As indicated above, robotics provides a unique opportunity to integrate all the functions of a surgical procedure (surgeon, assistant, nurse, etc.) into a single system. The next generation of robotics will also include entirely new capabilities: smart instruments, automatic functions, energy-directed therapy and MEMS, nano-, and biosurgery. Smart instruments are those that include sensors or diagnostic capabilities within the surgical instrument. Instruments, such as graspers, will have sensors that provide the sense of touch, at normal sensory levels as well as scaled to even microforce levels—beyond the level a normal human hand can feel. Other instruments, such as scalpels, will include various diagnostic sensors (Raman spectroscopy, hyperspectral analysis) that will be able to distinguish between healthy and malignant tissue [10]. In addition, instruments are becoming multifunctional and capable of performing entire tasks. The most typical example is the end-to-end anastomosis (EEA) stapler. Rather than dividing the intestines and hand sewing the two ends together, current practice is to divide the bowel, attach the stapler, and with one squeeze of the hand, perform a complete anastomoses, usually with a higher level of precision than hand sewing. There are other new tools becoming available, such as a number of methods for automatically creating a vascular anastomosis [11]. Analysis of a surgical procedure can be done by breaking down the entire procedure into a series of sequential smaller tasks; it is reasonable to expect that it would be possible to automate each of the individual steps, eventually integrating all the steps into a single autonomous procedure. Once the integration of a sequence of steps is achieved, it would only be logical to simulate or rehearse the entire procedure (on patient specific three-dimensional CT scan); this procedure can also be edited (delete all the errors, like editing a document on a word processor), and then export the perfected procedure, step by step, to the robotic system to perform the entire procedure automatically—under the close supervision of the surgeon, who could intervene at any time. This is the methodology used every day in the engineering community: automating a process and supervisory control. Since robotic systems currently available can perform tasks at 12 to 15 times the speed, with 10 to 20 times the

precision of humans, it could be speculated that once the surgeon has rehearsed and edited the procedure on the virtual person, the robotic system could perform the procedure in minutes instead of hours, with greater precision. More speculative is the coupling of the human thought process to controlling robotic systems. The brain–machine interface systems that are in today's laboratories permits monkeys to control a robotic arm simply by thinking, albeit it at a very rudimentary level [12, 13]. As this technology rapidly progresses, there has been speculation that it will be possible to simply think through a complex task such as surgery and have the robotic systems perform to precision. While clearly beyond any technology that will be implemented by the current generation of surgeons, some lesser variation of direct intellectual control of robotic systems may emerge. This speculation is supported through analogy to the implementation of clinical trials in quadriplegic patients using an implanted brain chip to control robotic manipulator motion.

To the practicing surgeon, this means that surgery may place more and more emphasis on intellectual and cognitive skills and less on manual skills. Crafting a surgical procedure may become more important than performing the procedure. As advanced technology provides more precise automatic instruments (and robotics) and better surgical planning tools, surgeons must learn to master these new systems (rather than ignore them) and learn how to best integrate them into a busy clinical practice.

17.10 Unconventional Surgery

Most of the discussion has focused upon variations on established surgical practices using instruments that are a modification of current surgical tools. There are a number of new technologies that are fundamentally different. One class of technologies is the energy-directed systems, which include some ablation technologies in use today, such as radiofrequency (RF), thermal (cryo or heat), laser, as well as those used by radiologists such as X-ray, proton beam, etc. A significant difference between radiological and surgical use of energy systems (X-ray, proton beam, etc.) is that radiologists usually discharge X-rays over large areas to kill massive amounts of tissue, whereas the surgical energy tools are used with precision (and usually hand held) for very specific localized effect. There are other parts of the electromagnetic spectrum that are being investigated as potential energy-directed surgical tools: microwave, millimeter wave, femtosecond lasers, HIFU [14], photodynamic, and photoinduction therapy. What all these have in common is that they replace the conventional mechanical instruments of scalpel, clamp, and stapler with precisely directed energy. Although some of these new technologies are handheld instruments, the majority of these energy-directed tools are (and will be) controlled with robotic systems to provide accuracy and safety.

A second class of unconventional surgical instrument is the micro- and nanoscale systems (microsystems are a thousand times smaller and nanosystems are a million times smaller than are current instruments). Like energy-directed systems and because of their small size, micro- and nanoscaled systems must be computer controlled. Some simple microsystems are being used for ophthalmology, otolaryngology, plastic, and neurological surgery, the most commonly employed is LASIK surgery. The experimentation now is on creating entire machines on a microscopic level: for microscale there are the microelectromechanical systems (MEMS), which are etched from silicon wafers, and for nanoscale there are assemblies of molecules into specific configurations to produce tiny machines that can enter the blood stream and cells. At the time of this writing, demonstration nanoengines have been created but not designed specifically for any medical application—in essence, proof of concept. How far these systems will proceed to the vision of miniature machines traveling through the body and blood stream as depicted in Isaac Asimov's *The Fantastic Voyage* [15] is yet to be seen.

The impact of these unconventional new technologies is not predictable, because their use signals a complete disruption in the practice of surgery. This change is best characterized as follows. Current surgical technologies are used to resect, remove, replace, and repair organs and tissues—structure and anatomy; the unconventional technologies will be implemented at the cellular and molecular levels—changing the basic biology (and possibly DNA itself) without changing the anatomy but inducing the repair at a biologic level. Hence the term *biosurgery* has been applied to indicate this fundamental change [16]. The challenges to practicing surgeons are even greater, since it will be necessary to keep abreast of advances not only in the practice of surgery, but also for the basic sciences of biology, engineering, and informatics, a monumental task.

17.11 Conclusion

The principle tenant of disruptive technologies is that a revolutionary change challenges core knowledge and practice, and requires the surgeon to reevaluate his or her practice in order to adapt to the change, frequently on less-than-complete information or proof. This past century, and especially the past 20 years, has produced repeated assault on many aspects of surgery: mini-mally invasive approach, robotics, surgical simulation, transplantation, and many more. No longer is change being slowly and methodically introduced one change at a time; rather, the surgeon is being buffeted from many sides at once. Interdisciplinary knowledge is required to keep up with these changes, a quite impossible task in lieu of the many other stresses to clinical practice. The traditional approach to life-long learning through occasional continuing medical education (CME) courses must be supplemented by self education through journals, Web-based education, and other information-based systems. Keeping abreast of the latest surgical technologies, techniques, and procedures will require more than a weekend course; it must include subsequent mentoring and proctoring until proficiency is obtained before incorporating the new technology into a surgeon's clinical practice. And outcomes must be documented to prove that the acquisition of new skills and procedures has been done safely. Finally, it is imperative for surgeons to carefully address the moral and ethical implications of the new technologies, to ensure that not only can it be introduced safely, but that the technology will not have unintended long-term consequences. The burden upon surgeons has never been so great.

References

1. Senn N (1908) The dawn of military surgery. Surgery, gynecology and obstetrics, pp 477–482
2. Giuliano KA, Haskins JR, Taylor DL (2003) Advances in high content screening for drug discovery. Assay Drug Dev Technol 1:565–577
3. Marescaux J, Clement JM, Tassetti V, Koehl C, Sotin S, Russier Y, Mutter D, Delingette H Ayache N (1998) Virtual reality applied to hepatic surgery simulation: the next revolution. Ann Surg 228:627–634
4. Altobelli DE, Kikinis R, Mulliken JB, Cline H, Lorensen W, Jolesz F (1993) Computer-assisted three dimensional planning in craniofacial surgery. Plastic Reconstruct Surg 92:576–585
5. Sandberg WS, Ganous TJ, Steiner C (2003) Setting a research agenda for perioperative systems design. Semin Laparosc Surg 10:57–70
6. Martin JA, Regehr G, Reznick R, MacRae H, Murnaghan J, Hutichinson C, Brown M (1997) Objective structured assessment of technical skill (OSATS) for surgical residents. Br J Surg 84:273–278
7. Derossis AM, Fried GM, Abrahamowicz M, Sigman HH, Barkun JS, Meakins JL (1998) Development of a model of evaluation and training of laparoscopic skills Am J Surg 175:482–487
8. Seymour NE, Gallagher AG, Roman SA, O'Brien MK, Bansal VK, Andersen D, Satava RM (2002) Virtual reality training improves operating room performance: results of a randomized, double-blinded study. Ann Surg 236:458–464

9. Lalan S, Pomerantsva I, Vacanti JP (2001) Tissue engineering and its potential impact on surgery. World J Surg 25:1458–1466

10. Verimetra, Inc. http://www.verimetra.com

11. Wolff R, Alderman EI, Caskey MP et al (2003) Clinical and six-month angiographic evaluation of coronary arterial graft interrupted anastomoses by use of self-closing clip device: A multicentrial prospective clinical trial. J Thorac Cardiovasc Surg 126:168–177

12. Serruya MD, Hatsopoulos NG, Paninski L, Fellows MR, Donoghue JP (2002) Instant neural control of movement signal. Nature 416:121–122

13. Donoghue JP (2002) Connecting cortex to machines: recent advances in brain interfaces. Nat Neurosci 5(Suppl):1085–1088

14. Vaezy S, Martin R, Keilman G, Kaczkowski P, Chi E, Yazaji E, Caps M, Poliachik C, Carter S, Sharar S, Comejo C, Crum L (1999) Control of splenic bleeding by using high-intensity ultrasound. J Trauma 47:521–525

15. Asimov I, Klement O, Kleiner H (1966) The fantastic voyage. Houghton Mifflin, Boston

16. Satava RM, Wolff R (2003) Disruptive visions: biosurgery. Surg Endosc 17:1833–1836

Subject Index